I0411085

Quieting the Chaos

Organizing Disorganized Thoughts

Louie Keyes

Grateful Wings Publishing

First printing

ISBN 978-1537516-3-87 (paperback)

Printed in the United States of America

~ written with my own children in mind and

the hope that all children will be cared for the way they should ~

Contents

Preface

I need groceries—that's my mission. I'm in my car, within a block of the grocery store. I see a red car. My thoughts shift. My mission shifts. The Force is calling. No, I need groceries. Stay on the task.

I resolutely put the Force out of my mind, but then a second red car crosses the intersection in front of me. This car is two tones, red and green. The added green must mean the Force wants me to see something special. I look wildly at the people walking and driving, at the colors of their clothing, the expressions on their faces, anything that might tell me what to do next. I look at the colors of the houses, their shapes and sizes, and any dogs and cats, squirrels and birds for a clue to my next move.

I try again to ignore the Force. The Force can both hurt me and protect me. I am afraid. I must find the message. I become more and more frantic as I can't locate what the Force is trying to tell me. Then I see another red car and know that means to stop. I pull over to park and wait for the Force to tell me what to do next. I need the Force to direct me where to go or not to go, something, anything.

Twenty minutes later, a blue and green car goes by. The green wants me to start driving again. Mentally and emotionally exhausted, I obey the signs and drive wherever they point the way. A brown and tan car goes by. I follow it. Another car goes by. I switch and follow that one. I notice a parked red car. Now red means I should change direction so I turn off at the next intersection. As I turn I see another car with red on it. I turn again and see a person walking wearing all blue. I look up at the sky to see if there's a message. I continue to drive, turning, turning again, following, and turning again. Finally, without groceries, I get back home.

▲▼▲▼▲

Hi. My name is Louie Keyes. Twenty-three years ago I entered a mental institution with a life sentence and a diagnosis of Acute Paranoid Schizophrenia (later changed to Paranoid Delusional–Persecutory Type). I was responsible for bringing unspeakable pain into the lives of the families and friends of the people I killed and into the lives of my own family and friends, too. In our community, I added to the general fear and anxiety that people feel when they feel powerless to keep themselves and their loved ones safe.

Once I was in the institution, the question I kept asking myself was, "What happened? What happened?" Actually, I knew *what* happened; what I didn't know was *how* I went from being an innocent child who grew up wanting to help others to being the kind of person who could kill someone. I wanted to try to trace my road to mental illness and to the crimes I committed. Later I realized that I wanted to build a new road to recovery. Initially I didn't have the language for that goal.

I sensed that if I didn't figure out what was going on with me, I could never trust what I would or wouldn't do. I might be medicated to the point that I would have no self left. I might be unable to spontaneously respond to my environment. Feeling lethargic and developing long-term health issues are possible side effects of the medications usually prescribed for my diagnosis. I might find myself depending on something external for control instead of developing my own self-control. My bewilderment about how I'd done what I did helped motivate me to take this journey of self-exploration. My health concerns and concerns about losing myself to the medications helped me find the courage to get started.

This is my story. I started writing it for myself and then started to wonder if others might be helped by it. Maybe it could help someone who has a friend or loved one struggling with mental illness. Maybe my story could help that someone understand what the world looks like to his friend or to her friend. Maybe it could help someone who is an aide or doctor helping people who have a mental illness. Maybe my story could help remind that someone that he or she and I are both strong and fragile, have good days and bad days, and that how we are treated makes a difference.

This story is not about my crime or my victims, except for what you will need to know so as to understand what it was like, what happened, and the healing I have experienced so far. The first seven chapters are about my life's events and trying to figure things out. In Chapter 8, I talk about what has helped and continues to help me stay healthy. I've also included a section at the end with some of my songs and poems, because I think they reveal a lot about me and my journey, and then there's a section of the outside resources, like books and movies, that helped and continue to help me.

With the exception of changing some names, places, and dates, the story is true. I hope my book helps you better understand someone you know.

Chapter 1

Life Begins

Back in the 60s a very popular TV series called *The Andy Griffin Show* came on weekly. It took place in a small town called Mayberry, and I could tell Mayberry was the type of town most everyone wanted to grow up in. Mayberry was beautiful with streets to stroll down and ride bikes on and where everyone knew everyone else and people cared about each other. They got into little troubles, but they got fixed in half an hour. People in Mayberry seemed happy and, most of all, safe.

I can see myself at age 4, Opie's age, waking up very early on a wintry morning and going to the kitchen window. Everyone else is still asleep. To my surprise the world is covered with snow and the big white flakes continue to fall from the dark gray sky. The snow is so heavy you can hardly see through it. The cars below are all but covered. I can feel the silence as nothing is moving. In that silence it's as if time has stopped. It feels peaceful, safe, and magical. No one is around to hurt me in any way. I didn't realize then that feeling safe and peaceful seemed imaginary to me. I believe in hell. For me it was a place where I lived in constant fear, but didn't know it. It's a place where I was learning to trust no one, especially myself, but I didn't know it. In my hell, sometimes people are afraid to think, afraid to talk, afraid to move, and then at times afraid to breathe. I thought hell was supposed to be a place for adults, but there I was only 4 years old and in hell, but I didn't know it. My unconscious inner plea was, "Dad, Mom, please! Help me! What am I supposed to do? What am I supposed to say?" The tears come and the fear remains. I became afraid of being nobody and terrified of being somebody.

I was born in the spring of 1943. For the first ten years of my life, we lived in a tiny three-room apartment house in Chicago, Illinois. There were seven of us in my family—Mom, Dad, and then in order, an older sister, an older brother, me, and two younger sisters.

Dad moved out when I was four. Was he still at home when I was looking out the window at the snow? Did I feel that sense of safety and peace because I knew he was there or because I knew he was gone? I don't remember. I remember Mom holding onto Dad's arm as he was trying to leave the house. He pushed her off and left. Mom sat down at the table where my two younger sisters and I were also sitting as we witnessed the scene. Mom put her head down on her arms and cried. I was very sad. After that Dad popped in and out sometimes, but he lived somewhere else.

As a family, we didn't function well. We learned early on in life that you don't talk about problems or express feelings like fear, hurt, anger, or sadness. Questions and statements like, "How are you?" "I love you!" and "How was your day?" were unheard of. The closest we saw how healthy families functioned was by watching TV programs, like *Father Knows Best*, *Ozzie and Harriet*, and *Leave It to Beaver*. These programs were important because I could escape from my fears into the worlds of Springfield, Hollywood Hills, and Mayberry and be the various characters. Watching these programs gave me a sense of hope and amazement.

I never really felt a part of my family back then, but I desperately wanted to. In my head I was responding with an angry, "Who cares anyway!" but underneath it sounded more like a plea, "Please help me! Does anyone out there care?" The main reason I did not feel a part of my family is because I didn't feel like I had any value. The brutal beatings I received at such a young age from my father did the most damage and set the stage for me to not accept or value myself. Being in the formative years of my life and being severely hurt on both a physical and emotional level by the ones I loved and depended on the most sent a very powerful message. That message said something was wrong with me. I knew it must be true. Sometimes my siblings would not play with me because my older brother told them not to. They would say, "You stink" or "Get away from me." I know other kids get called names, and I guess I was a more sensitive child than most. Or maybe all kids feel the same way. I don't know. I don't remember my mom talking to me much at all.

I'm guessing each of my siblings experienced something different. In talking with my oldest sister I know she didn't get along with Mom, and my brother didn't get along with Dad. I am not sure how things were for my next younger sister. My youngest sister seemed to be treated the best. I only know we were all affected by the dysfunction of our family, and we were all in need of love. I suppose our parents didn't know how to give us the love that they themselves did not receive.

First Memories

I have fond memories of playing in the piled up snow on the curbs after the snowplows came through, climbing on the pile like mountains, making snowmen, and having snowball fights with the neighborhood kids. During a good rain, I pulled on my yellow rain slicker and hat and raced boats with my friend in the rainwater rushing down the slope of our street. We used little wooden Popsicle sticks for our boats. We took the race very serious as we ran alongside our imaginary boats, sometimes arguing over whose stick belonged to whom. I think these are my first memories of feeling freedom of expression. I knew then that it was important to me.

On one such occasion, after reaching the bottom of the hill, we started arguing about who won. I saw a flattened beer can with mud on it along the curb. I picked it up and slung it towards him hitting him square in the face. He started crying and went home. The accuracy of my throw surprised me and felt good. It was like

I did something right but in the same moment it frightened me because I could have seriously hurt him. I deeply regretted hurting a friend like that.

Christmas was the best holiday by far. It brought the warmest and greatest feelings ever. What will Santa bring this year? There was no doubt in my mind that there was a Santa Claus. Because there was no fireplace for Santa to come down the chimney, I wondered how all that was going to work. I figured Santa probably landed his sleigh on the roof and used the back porch door to get in. I could imagine Mom paying Santa for the gifts, putting them under the tree, and then going back to bed.

The anticipation and excitement of Santa coming and the whole Christmas feel was so wonderful. No school, the buying of the Christmas tree, decorating it, the nuts, cookies, various candies, Christmas music, the snow, the presents, and of course Christmas Eve, the day before the big event. All these things and more played a part in making it the perfect time. The climax was waking up, seeing the presents, and opening them. One year I might get those little green army men along with a filling station and cars. As I got a little older, it was a six-shooter that uses caps to make it seem real. When I discovered that Mama was Santa, I tried not to let her find out that I knew because I didn't want her to feel sad.

I really loved my mom and missed her when she went to work. Mom was a strict disciplinarian. Under very challenging circumstances, she raised five kids with very little help. She worked very hard to make ends meet, working both a full and a part-time job for over twenty years. My great grandmother babysat us. She made the best cornbread that we dipped in buttermilk. Even in her 80s my great grandma was feisty. When I got out of line, she grabbed one of my ears and slowly started twisting it. As her twisting intensified, so did my whining, getting louder and higher in pitch like a fire truck siren. Hers was the first funeral that I attended. Being at the funeral home and seeing her in the casket, I knew I would never see her again. It was so quiet with sad music playing. I didn't cry until I got home and was by myself.

Because Mom worked so much, I saw very little of her. When she was home, she was busy cooking and taking care of things around the house. Conversation was scarce and hugs were nonexistent. I cannot say enough about my mom's cooking. It was the best. She cooked bacon and eggs, made cakes, pies, hot rolls, and biscuits, homemade ice cream, roast, chicken, turkey, hamburgers, cheeseburgers, French fries, beans, oatmeal, rice, and peanut butter and jelly sandwiches. You name it and my mom could make it, bake it, or cook it.

As I reflect on these early memories, in spite of everything, both mom and my grandmother were in my life and at that time gave me my first impressions of what it was like to feel safe and cared for. I love them for that. A part of me longs for and misses that caring and feeling of safety they gave.

Playing with the Neighborhood Kids

We lived in an isolated section of town that was called "The Hills." It was like a little bitty city within a city. There were three very small mom-and-pop grocery stores, three bars, and one restaurant. Behind the neighborhood, two hills each had a set of long concrete steps to get in or out of the neighborhood where we played. Our neighborhood was famous for having a company called Red Yeast. Sometimes you could smell the yeast from far away.

Across the street from our house, there were railroad tracks instead of houses. A passenger train called the Hiawatha raced past day and night. Our house vibrated from the clickity-clack. Some trains were transportation trains loaded with new cars, trucks, and tractors. Others were who-knows-what and cattle cars. One time the cows escaped, and railroad workers were running around with ropes trying to catch them. It was a sight to see.

I did a lot of risky things with my brother and the neighborhood kids when I was about 6 to 10 years old. Sometimes when a long, slow moving train came by, we kids actually jumped on it and rode it for a little ways. Although aware, we weren't discouraged by the fact a serious injury or sudden death awaited us if a mistake was made.

When we played follow-the-leader—usually one of the older kids—we had to do whatever the leader did or we'd be out the game. If the leader climbed onto the roof of a two-story house and jumped across to the roof of the next house, we were supposed to jump, too. I was too little to do that. One of the older girls broke her leg. Another dangerous game that we played was to go on top of the first hill behind the houses and roll tires down on unsuspecting cars driving down the street. The driver sometimes jumped out of the car and ran up the hill chasing us, but by the time he got on top of the first hill, we were on top of the second hill laughing.

One of my most intriguing memories of fun adventures was playing on top of an old two-story garage. The garage roof was completely torn off leaving the inside exposed to the elements. The second story floor was intact with the roof's support beams sticking up into the air. It looked like a fort with turrets back in the days of the knights. Some of us played the good guys in the fort while others played the bad guys trying to take the fort. A few times a week we gathered for our war games but not without risk.

The garage was owned by an old man we called Dynamite Twig, who also owned the neighborhood mom-and-pop grocery store. You'd be lucky to fit ten people in the store at one time. I liked him. I think his last name might have been Weaver. When we kids stopped in to buy candy, Dynamite waited on us never saying one word.

While in the heat of battle over the ruined garage, Dynamite Twig had a habit of suddenly appearing out of nowhere and throwing rocks at us still never saying a word. Someone would yell, "Dynamite Twig!" and we'd all take off running. Dynamite chased us a few feet and then he went back to the store. We stayed away a bit until we considered it "safe" and then headed back to the fort and sooner or later out came Dynamite throwing those rocks again. He could care less about who were the good guys or bad—Dynamite Twig threw those rocks at all of us. While we were playing we even went into the store from time to time to buy his candy. He never said anything about us playing on his garage. It was like he was playing his part in our fantasy games.

Dynamite Twig and the fort really stand out for me. I think it's because there we all were misbehaving and, except for me stepping on a rusty nail one time, no one got hurt. No way could I have had that kind of fun with my dad. I think Dynamite was the dad who didn't hurt me or carry a grudge. I will always cherish and never forget this strange and at the same time beautiful relationship with Dynamite Twig.

Probably the most dangerous thing we did was on the ten-story high 53rd Street Bridge. It was a very long bridge and one of several bridges that connected the south and north sides of town. Long steps led to the top of the bridge and onto a narrow walk. Just under the walk near the very top was a narrow wooden plank that spanned the whole bridge. Us kids walked across that plank. Below it were the train tracks and a small lake.

On some nights, encouraged by my older brother who was only 12 years old himself, my brother and I not only climbed up on that dangerous plank, we climbed from that plank onto the support rails of the bridge to catch baby pigeons. As frightened as

I was, climbing that bridge gave me a great sense of accomplishment. And, I wanted my big brother to be proud of me.

We made a home for the pigeons in a big cage we built behind the house. We kept the cage clean and fed the pigeons hard kernels of corn and gave them fresh water every day. We also fed them small rocks that helped with their digestion. One day, when the pigeons were grown, we made the decision to let them go. We opened the cage door. One by one they flew out onto the roof of our house. Everyone thought that was the end of it. To our surprise, when evening came, they flew back into the cage, one by one just like airplanes. To the pigeons, that *was* their home.

Not everything we did was risky. I enjoyed pretend camping on the first hill with the Kool-Aid and sandwiches we brought along. Sometimes we saw deer, and there were lots of rabbits and squirrels. Picnics at Bell Park across the bridge included watching the fish in the pond, boating, and swimming. Trips to State Fair Park were a special adventure. Five dollars got you there and back on the bus, lots of rides, and a meal back in those days. Sometimes they paid kids to help them break down the rides at the end of summer. We started just after midnight and worked until daybreak.

After writing this the tears came. These were some of the most exciting times of my life. I had fun, and I felt alive with excitement. I felt a part of something with others, and I felt accepted. I felt loved.

Although Dad no longer lived with us, he left a lot of his things at the house. Probably most important to me was an extensive music collection. Music was soothing and beautiful to my ear. Music became important at a young age. Waiting for Mom to come home so we could go out—one of the family rules—I listened to music on Dad's records and the radio and listened to radio shows and watched TV. I liked *Howdy Doody* and westerns like *The Roy Rogers and Dale Evans Show*, *Hopalong Cassidy*, *The Lone Ranger*, *Cisco Kid*, and, of course, *Superman.* I became the characters. I was always the good guy. Helping and saving people from the villains. I had a purpose. I mattered. I had value. I was worthy. Like the shows, the flow and melodies and vocal harmonies of the music took me to a whole new world. It was like getting a message after a hard day's work to not be afraid or worry about pain or problems. When I heard Pat Boone sing *Friendly Persuasion,* I imagined myself on a flying carpet high above the ground feeling ever so safe and totally free. Even in this moment I can feel that freedom. It brings a smile to my face.

The Neighborhood House

I spent a lot of happy hours at a summer and after-school camp called The Neighborhood House. It didn't start off happy though. I was in the 5 to 7-year-olds group. Being shy and not talking much was a pattern for me then. I didn't play or talk with the other kids. The counselors tried but couldn't get me to open up. One day, my group gathered all our lunches and swimming trunks on a little hill in bushel baskets. The counselor and kids headed off somewhere, and I stayed behind, alone on the hill. I later overheard a counselor named Jane tell the story of what happened next. The other counselors could see me on the hill. One moment they looked up and I was just sitting there on one of the picnic tables. The next moment they looked up and saw me throwing everyone's stuff from the bushel baskets all over the hill. One of the counselors named Ray told the other counselors to just leave me alone. After that I started talking again. I remember this as a rare time when I freely expressed my anger and was not punished for it.

During the winter months, my older brother and sister and I raced and dodged street traffic to The Neighborhood House as soon as school let out. The counselors greeted us at the front door like they were glad to see us. We played games, wrestled, did crafts, sang songs, and watched movies. One time my brother and some of his friends were in the talent show. While singing a song, they accompanied themselves by slapping their legs and chests with open hands creating a cool sounding beat. This type of accompaniment is called the *ham bone*. Their performance made a huge impression on me and motivated me to want to do something like that. I wanted to impress people, too. And it was just a cool thing to witness their talents.

I remember one bad experience I had at The Neighborhood House. It was the end of the day and we were coming back from one of the parks. I fell asleep at the back of the bus. All of a sudden I was awakened by one of the councilors slapping my face. I didn't know what was happening and was very scared. I never told anyone. I was feeling so safe. It was like home. It was a reminder to me that I wasn't safe anywhere.

In 1953, I was 6 years old, and it was my second year attending The Neighborhood House summer camp. The yellow school bus, mostly driven by Ray, took us to different parks around the city. A new counselor we called Blondie was the counselor for my age group. She was nice and pretty and I liked her about as much as a six-year-old could like anybody. One day as the yellow bus took us to a new park, we passed a spot I recognized from when Dad took us kids fishing. Then we passed a famous area landmark called the Fruit Ranch. The Fruit Ranch stood out because it only had a roof with open sides. Blondie said, "I live out here." We were about three miles from my home.

As the summer came to an end, I was feeling sad. Blondie had made that summer so very special, and I probably would never see her again. The next day, as my friend Michael and I played together, I said, "Let's go find Blondie." Michael liked Blondie, too, so off we went.

It's not like we had any idea where Blondie lived, just that she lived near the Fruit Ranch. We didn't have any directions or a street name or an address, but we were determined to find her anyway. After crossing a long bridge and walking a mile or so, we finally reached the Fruit Ranch. After a few blocks walking in the same direction the bus had gone, a car turned down a street, so we decided to turn down that street, too. I knocked on the door of one of the houses and said to the man who answered, "We're looking for a lady named Blondie who works at a place called The Neighborhood House." He said he didn't know her.

We continued down the street and saw a man raking leaves and again I said, "We're looking for a lady named Blondie who worked at a place called The Neighborhood House with kids." The man said that his neighbor down the street had a daughter home from school and she was blonde and she worked with kids somewhere.

Our anticipation grew as we approached the house. I rang the doorbell and through the screen door we could see Blondie heading towards us. The feeling I experienced could not have been better than finding heaven. With surprise she opened the door and said, "How did you get here?" We said, "We walked." She was so nice. She invited us in and gave us milk and cookies. We watched TV while she was running around doing things. We were content. What were the odds of finding the right house? A little later she drove us home.

My journey to find Blondie and The Neighborhood House experience brought a big, big smile to my face and made me laugh as I wrote about it. I learned to take chances. I also learned what it felt like—wonderful!—to be with people you feel accepted by.

My Dad

When Dad came around, he mostly aimed to be alone. He always seemed to be very serious. To see him laugh or smile was rare. Later in my life, knowing this helped me understand where some of my own ways came from. In a rare instance of fathering, Dad said if a man had one friend, he's lucky. He said he had three. I never saw much of his friends. The few I met seemed nice and likeable. They treated me like they liked me, which was very different than what I experienced from my dad.

Dad loved to fish. Even though Mom and Dad were separated, sometimes he stopped by and took us all fishing. One of the fishing spots we went to was on a farmer's land that he knew. Sometimes we stayed overnight, and Dad set up a big green army tent with two sleeping cots for the adults. Us kids slept in the car. The farmer had lots of cows and one morning we woke up to find cows all around the car with their noses pressed against the window looking curiously at us, as if the cows were visiting us in a zoo instead of the other way around. Once out of the car, we chased the cows and the cows chased us.

I have a very clear memory picture of us camping and Mom cooking on a small gas stove with the wonderful smell of bacon and eggs infusing the air. Dad fished with his rod and reel or used a *setline*. A setline is a long thick rope with lots of hooks as big as your hand strung out all along it. After Dad baited all the hooks with some smelly stuff called catfish bait, he strung the rope out across the river and left it. After some time passed, he pulled it in and there were huge catfish on it, some as tall as we were. I don't have too many memories of all of us together as a family doing something fun and exciting, but this is one.

On some days Dad came and woke me up early in the morning before daylight to go fishing. It was rare. He didn't have the skills to talk to me and ask me things like, "How are you?" or "What's going on in your life?" He was very quiet and mostly just ordered me around. Still, it was just me and my dad. I felt special. He chose me. Writing this brought tears.

Dad had another side to him, a brutal side. There was no way to predict which side was going to show up. When I was around 4 years old, I was warned about keeping my shoes tied. One day Dad came home and saw that my shoes were untied again. He very calmly told me to go in and take off my clothes. I started crying and pleading to give me another chance. He usually beat me with a belt, ironing cord, or a thin, small, flexible tree branch. Because I was little, Dad could grab me by one leg and hold me in the air with one arm while beating me with the other. The pain was intense, and I yelled and struggled desperately and begged for another chance. As he kept beating me, he kept telling me to shut up. When he was done, he left without saying a word. Dad beat me for untied shoes, for playing in the backyard dirt, and for getting a bad report card. He called me dumb when I couldn't name all of the Great Lakes. Worse than the beatings was sitting in that big chair naked waiting to be beaten. One time I sat in the chair so long—naked and afraid—I fell asleep. When I woke up, Dad was gone. That was a miracle day.

Just one hurtful word or action can impact a child in a negative way for a lifetime. I felt so much terror; I felt so all alone; I felt so trapped. I was reduced to shame. It killed some of my spirit. I became suspicious and distrustful.

Sometimes I didn't see Dad for months at a time, and then he would just appear out of nowhere for a few hours and then he was gone again. I didn't know if I wished for more of his presence and more of his time or if I wished he would stay away because of his erratic nature and his beatings. I felt more and more alone, isolated, and angry.

At about age 8, I had a nightmare in which I took a human life. At the time I didn't know who it was or for what reason I'd do such a thing. I only remember someone was trying to hurt me in some way. I awoke from the dream sweating in a panic. I was terrified. Once I realized it was just a dream, I felt euphoric with gratitude.

In another recurring dream, I was in the backyard late at night all by myself. The neighbor's yard next door had turned into a small lake. I had this sense that some kind of monster was in it, and the monster was going to come out to get me at any moment. I ran and opened the hallway door that led upstairs to my house. Instead of running up the stairs, I was in such a panic I stopped and hid behind the door. I was hoping that if the monster came in, it would continue up the stairs and while it was upstairs I could run back out and get away. The door slowly opened, in came the monster and started up the stairs, but after a few steps it stopped, turned around, and saw me. As it was reaching down to get me, I woke up terrified.

Sometimes in the dreams I could get away from danger by being super fast. Other times it felt like weights were on my legs. One time I was able to float upright into the air. It felt so good and safe. I was able to fly in quite a few of my dreams. Sometimes, I struggled to get off the ground as an adversary was closing in on me.

I felt increasingly helpless and worthless, and my low self-esteem had an effect on my hygiene. I stopped combing my hair and taking baths. I began having nervous conditions and started picking the skin off my lips until they bled. I have since wondered if that was related to being told to shut up while being beaten. Other kids didn't want to play with me. I didn't know what to call it then, but I knew something was not right with me. It left me feeling empty and unconsciously searching and trying to find ways to eliminate that emptiness.

Watching TV, especially war movies, was one way I tried to fill that emptiness inside me. I identified with the good guys and when something bad happened to them, I went to bed sobbing and wishing I could have been there to save or help them. Even though it was TV, it still felt so real. Looking back, the crying was probably also about wishing someone cared enough about me to want to come and rescue me from my own hell. There was no escape.

Moving

When I was going on 10 years old, we moved to a different part of town. It was the last thing I wanted to do! It was heading into the unknown. To be leaving behind the first and only house I had ever known, the first neighborhood I had ever known, people I knew, and school, the railroad tracks, the 53rd Street Bridge, Bell Park, and a very special place called The Neighborhood House was scary. I could count on these things to be there, things that brought joy and excitement into my life. Not pain.

The new house was a single three-bedroom house instead of a three-room apartment. My brother and I had our first bedroom and bunk beds instead of a rollaway bed in the kitchen. I was surprised when it turned out that I did like some things about the new house.

School

I remember how scary the first day of school was. Outside of my brother and sister who took me there, I didn't know anyone. I wasn't used to being around so many people for such a long time. So much was happening and it was all so new that one of my first days of school I couldn't find the classroom so I went back outside and sat on the school steps until lunchtime. Then I went home with a little boy who I didn't even know. I got in trouble for that.

Some good things happened to me in school before things got bad. In the sixth grade I played end on the tag football team. Mr. Schuler was the coach and one of my teachers. He was very, very strict. No one messed with Mr. Schuler. We were going to play the 21st Street School and everyone was talking about their best player, a defender named Jake.

The game was winding down. Our team had the ball but we were losing by one point. It was the last play of the game, and it was ours to lose or win. The play was called in the huddle. I was to go down the line from the left, turn in, and receive the ball. When the quarterback called the last hut, I took off, turned in, and the pass was in the air. If I didn't catch the ball and score, the game was over. I caught the ball and ran as fast as I could with Jake in hot pursuit. I could hear him closing in, and it looked like Jake was going to catch me.

Playing with regular shoes on was slowing me down, but I ran like I did back in the old neighborhood on The Hills when the drivers stopped and chased us for rolling tires down on them or when I ran away from Dynamite Twig. I crossed the line and *touchdown*! It was an awesome feeling, but I showed very little emotion on the outside when the team surrounded me. Mr. Schuler was beaming with pride. We had just beaten the feared 21st Street School. I was fully accepted. I was a hero. It was so special. Things people dream about came true for me on that day.

Chapter 2

Adolescence

At thirteen we moved again. I met a guy named Jimmy and we became very good friends. Jimmy went to church on Sundays where he was a junior deacon. He was sometimes asked to say a prayer with the whole congregation listening. I thought that was pretty cool. He invited me to become a junior deacon, so I started attending meetings and soon I became one, too. I think of Jimmy as a faithful friend even to this day.

After attending church regularly for some months, something happened that I felt was not right. A man who everyone at the church looked up to became involved with a married lady. I became disillusioned about church and God and quit. It wasn't until much later in my life that I realized that when I gave up on God as well as that church, I was throwing the baby out with the bathwater. I felt lost and began my search for something meaningful again.

A few years went by without any beatings but that was about to change.

There would be only two more beatings. For the first time, a friend of mine saw it. I don't remember what we did but as Jimmy told me the story he said he never saw anyone get beat like that before. He said he thought my dad was trying to kill me. Jimmy said he ran because he assumed he would be next. I was stunned when Jimmy told me what he saw because I can't even remember it.

I was getting nothing but bad report cards. Mom was upset about the latest report card, and Dad just happened to come by the house. Talk about bad timing. He hadn't been by in months. I knew I was in big trouble, so I headed to my room, closed the door, got into bed and pulled the covers over me pretending to be asleep. Dad threw open the door and snatched the blankets off me. Having the bottom bunk unfortunately made for easier access.

Wailing on me with his belt, I started hollering. As he was beating me, he kept saying over and over, again and again, "Are–you–going–to–pass? Are–you–going–to–pass?" He said it in this steady, rhythmic way. I kept hollering over and over, "I'm–going–to–pass. I'm–going–to–pass." It seemed like it went on forever. Finally Mom came in and said to Dad, "Honey, you know you have a bad heart."

He stopped and left the room. Laying there crying, I heard Mom talking to him. She said, "I'm going to the store and will be right back." She went down the stairs and when the downstairs door closed, the bedroom door swung open and Dad started beating me again. "Are–you–going–to–pass? Are–you–going–to–pass?" "I'm–going–to–pass. I'm–going–to–pass." It didn't matter what I said. The beating would have been worse, but the top bunk restricted his swing. That was the last beating. Instead of making me do better in school, it made me even more sure that I was worthless.

As the years went by, the unresolved buried pain and fear became so deep that it felt like death. My anger and rage grew to frighten even me. Because of my pain and anger, I understood and identified with people who randomly started killing innocent people. I still recognized, however, that those were not the actions of someone who cared for people. I thought about the wars and hatred throughout the world that people had for one another regarding religion, race, lust for power, and greed. I wished for peace and couldn't understand why there couldn't be peace just as easily as there were wars.

I had so many questions about myself and about life: "Who am I?" "Where do I belong?" "Who wants me around?" "Where will I be accepted?" "Was I from another planet?" "Is what I am looking for over here?" "Is it over there?" "What do I have to do to find happiness?" "Do I have to do this?" "Do I have to do that?" "Was money the answer?" "Is having a girlfriend or wife the answer?" "Where is happiness?" "Where is peace?" "What is the truth?" "Is there a God?" "What is God?" "Where is God?" "What is love?" "Where is love?" "What does it mean to love?" Happiness became something I learned to fear. It felt dangerous to feel happy. It just wasn't safe. I felt desperate to understand.

Seventh Grade

In seventh grade, I attended South High School until the new junior high school was built. Most of my grades were failing grades. I met some new guys in seventh grade and became a person whose greatest aim is to please people. I goofed off all the time, clowned around with my friend, got high, and skipped classes. Hanging with Bob, my best friend, gave me status because Bob was known and liked by most all the kids. Around Bob I was kind of quiet because Bob was the show. One of the big differences between the guys and me was when it came time to do homework—they did theirs and I didn't.

The first time I got high was with Colt 45 malt liquor. I started drinking wine and then whiskey. Eventually pills, like Red Devils. They made you feel drunk. Then there was speed, marijuana, and cough syrup. I tried cocaine and didn't like it. I thought about heroin but didn't like needles. All the time I was doing this, there was a part of me that didn't like any of it.

At first getting high was to be cool with those I was hanging with. An additional benefit was it muted my feelings of insecurity, and that's when it started to become even more of a problem. It was no longer necessary to be around the guys any more to get high.

For the school variety show, I put a little singing group together. Clancy was lead singer, and I sang background harmonies. Music helped me to start backing away from getting high and putting some distance between me and the guys I had been hanging out with. Our group became one of the top groups in the area. Whenever the YMCA had a dance, we could be counted on to sing. Our vocal harmony was great, and we sounded as good as any group on the radio.

I met a girl named Mary, and we liked each other a lot. When with the old gang, if a girl showed any interest in me, they would say, "Why don't you get some of that?" My response was, "There's more to it than just sex." They just shook their heads. When Mary and I started going steady, one of the guys in the singing group said they were going to throw me a party when I finally kissed her. I really liked Mary's mother and siblings, and they liked me, too. Mary's mother and father were also separated, which gave us something in common. I felt Mary and her family truly liked me and that was a whole new experience.

High School

Because of my involvement with music, drugs continued to fade out of the picture. Sports began to interest me so I tried out for wrestling in ninth grade. I found out the hard way that it was one of the most physically strenuous sports there was to do. On the first day of practice, the coach paired us up to show what we could do. I threw my teammate all around the mat and then ran out of gas and lost. My luck was much better with the second guy, but after practice I was so worn out that getting dressed was a real struggle. Staggering all the way home, I vowed to never return. Watching the same guy who beat me in practice get demolished by the state champ at a meet from the stands was just fine with me.

My cousin was the state champ in the 100- and 200-yard dash so I thought, why not try for track. I chose the 440-yard race. I had one little problem though and that was always goofing off during practice. If the girls were watching the pole-vaulters, I was with the pole-vaulters. If the girls were watching the 100-yard dash, there I was with the 100-yard dashers.

The guy who normally ran the 440 was sick the day of the meet against Thomas High School. After a few of the guys advocated strongly to the coach for me to run, the coach, said, "Okay, Louie, you're going to run."

When the gun sounded, I took off like I was running the 100-yard dash. I heard the girls say, "Wow! Who is that?" Coming around the first bend, my legs started tightening up, and I started slowing down. One runner passed, then another. I had nothing left in the tank. After such an explosive, impressive start, there was no way I wanted to be last. The final runner came up alongside me. We were neck and neck for the last few feet. As we reached the finish line, I stuck my chest out liked the professionals and fell flat on my face. Dead last and so exhausted, I had to be helped off the field. The lesson learned from that was easy. "No practice, no win."

Music

My oldest sister became a nurse and an attorney. My brother became a teacher, and the sister next youngest to me worked for a judge. They have since retired. My youngest sister retired from the Navy and became a teacher, too. A career in music was my goal and my passion.

At seventeen, music was one of the few things I took seriously. Being the leader of the four or at times five-man singing group was all business. If someone wasn't on time for practice, they heard about it. A more mature Louie began to develop.

Dad had once told me that if I ever needed something to let him know ahead of time. The high school variety show was coming up and my singing group was going to perform. We decided to wear suits. With the show about a month away, Dad happened to stop by the house and I let him know that I needed a new suit for the variety show. He said okay.

As the date of the show drew closer, there was no dad to be found. On the very day of the show, Dad drove up. Feeling relieved was putting it lightly. He came into the house but said nothing about the suit. It appeared that he just happened to stop by. I reminded him of the suit and he became agitated. Luckily, one of my sisters intervened on my behalf and reminded Dad of his promise. Once in his car to go get the suit, Dad angrily said,

"As long as you live, don't you ever ask me for anything again." I didn't say a word. My own father was saying to me, his son, "I don't want you in my life period."

Our performance was another success. The audience really liked us. I was sort of used to my own parents not being there. When school let out for the summer, the group continued to practice and performed little shows from time to time, like the YMCA dances. Mostly we did a lot of street corner singing. Sometimes some of the tougher guys in the area that we knew and got along with saw us coming down the street and made us sing a song before we could pass by them. We enjoyed doing it.

School was out for summer vacation, and one day, while listening to the radio, a great song came on that I had never heard. Most of the songs we covered called for a lead voice in the higher range that was popular back then. The lead vocalist for this song sang in a lower register, more like my voice. I practiced and practiced until I felt ready to sing it for the group. A few of the notes were high and hard to hit, but overall I felt good about how well it was going. At the next practice, I was ready to spring my surprise on the group. As I began to sing, our two lead singers busted out laughing. To cover up the embarrassment and pain I was feeling at their reaction, I laughed, too. This was a defining moment. I thought to myself, "I must be crazy for thinking that I could be a lead singer." Although disappointed, I knew the group recognized my abilities singing background vocals and so I remained confident when singing harmonies. Eventually the group broke up.

When I sang a song and people complimented me and seemed to mean it, I still found it hard to believe. I presently still struggle with that a little bit, but it feels good to have much more confidence than I had.

Chapter 3

On My Own

Still in high school, again alcohol and drug consumption began to increase. After waking up one morning from a night of alcohol and drugs, I couldn't remember how I got home or what I did. It frightened me. That had never happened before. It didn't stop me from drinking though. Mom was getting tired of me not following her rules. One night after coming home drunk about 2:00 AM, while fumbling around trying to get the key into the door, it opened and there she stood. She turned me around and told me I couldn't stay there. I stayed at a friend's house that night. That was the first time I had ever been thrown out of the house.

The next day I found another buddy to stay with. Things were not good. After a few weeks, I went home and asked Mom to give me another chance. She did. I was so glad.

Mom kept telling me how much I reminded her of my dad. That seemed strange because Dad did not drink. When I was younger, family members said that I was going to be just like my

Uncle Henry, an alcoholic. I didn't even drink at the time. I still don't understand the connection they saw.

One day Mom did something extremely unusual. She decided to go out of state to visit a relative for a few days. She told me not to have any of my friends over while she was gone. She reminded me that I had two younger sisters. By then my oldest sister was married, and my brother was in the military. Anyway, I told her I understood. No guys in the house while she was gone.

She couldn't have been gone no more than an hour, and I was on the phone calling up my friends letting them know that Mom was out of town and that they should come on over. There I was trying to impress the guys again. They had alcohol and marijuana. Taking it one step further, I told them they could stay overnight. They were sleeping all over the house, even in Mom's bed.

The next morning came. I was looking out the window. A cab pulled up in front of the house. Out stepped the last person I wanted to see—Mom. She was not supposed to come home for another two days. In a panic, I threw everyone out of the house but it was too late. She was furious, and I was thrown out of the house for good that morning.

I tried to act like it didn't bother me. I had to start learning what it was really like to be on my own—to have to find a place to live, pay the bills, find a job, keep a job, find transportation, upkeep it, and buy food and clothing. I started to see that love does not mean that there are no limits.

I ended up getting my own apartment. I was 18 years old at the time and, I must say, a very immature 18-year-old. My first night in my own apartment was scary. There I was in the dark for the very first time all by myself, looking for the boogieman. The next morning I made breakfast and went to school.

The school semesters went by, and my grades did not improve. I was still the class clown, feeling good when I could make people laugh. When graduation day came, I hid. I was so embarrassed. All my clowning buddies were graduating without me. The next semester came, and there I was, alone. School was never the same. I still showed up but rarely attended any scheduled classes. On two occasions, Mr. Patrick, the vice principal, suspended me after having given me several breaks.

One school morning out of boredom, I decided to give an unauthorized assembly program. Kids were waved out of the hallway into the assembly room. After gathering about ten people, I took the stage as the announcer and introduced a singer all the way from Italy. I went behind the curtain and came back out onstage and began to sing. I played all parts with the students laughing and laughing until Mr. Patrick showed up. All the students jumped up and ran for the exits. That was it for me. The goofing off, missing classes, bad grades, prior suspensions, and not graduating were too much for the school. Mr. Patrick expelled me. Even though I said, "I don't care," when he told me, I was at a loss as to what to do with my life. Half determined to get a high school diploma, I decided to attend vocational school. That didn't last long. I ended up dropping out. This was the end of something important that I still can't quite put into words and the beginning of even more serious stuff.

Military Service

It was 1966, and the Vietnam War was going strong. I decided to join the Marines. Maybe they could straighten me out. Nothing was working for me at home. There was just one failure after another. It became so tiresome. I wanted to make something out of my life and was desperate for some type of success. Mary, my girlfriend, was not happy when I broke the news.

I arrived in San Diego, California, late in the night and boarded a military bus. We headed to a military base called Camp Pendleton. Everything seemed okay at that point. On the way, no words were spoken to anyone. When we arrived at the base, we were rushed off the bus and told to get in a straight line. That's when things started to change. From a building nearby, a military man who was a sergeant approached us.

He stood in front of us all and very sternly shouted out that he was going to be our father, mother, brother, and sister. If we understood we were told to yell out, "Yes, sir!" We were then rushed off to another building for military haircuts. We all started looking more alike. With us all bald-headed, it was hard to recognize some of the guys. Then we turned in our street clothes for green fatigues. Next we got our bedding. Then we headed to our living quarters. This has all been awhile, so I'm trying to remember it the best that I can.

The first morning we were awakened around 4:00 AM very rudely by a man yelling and screaming at us to get out of the bed and to get outside where we started doing exercises. He was the drill instructor. We were constantly being yelled at. Then we marched over to eat.

I was starting to wonder if I had made a mistake. After all I was a volunteer. Why was all this rudeness necessary? It seemed to be about breaking you down, control, discipline, and handling pressure. It still didn't set well with me. I don't think it would with most people. We were cleaning our rifles one day, and I found myself thinking about home and wishing I was a stamp on an envelope. I could be home in a few days.

We were broken up into platoons consisting of forty or more men. A platoon was broken down into squads of about ten men each. I was chosen by the drill instructor as a squad leader. There were quite a few men older than me but I did okay. On the rifle range, depending on how well you hit the target in front of you, you became a marksman, sharpshooter, or expert. I was a sharpshooter.

When boot camp ended, there were about six or seven men out of the whole platoon promoted from private to private first class, also known as a Pfc. It was considered an honorary promotion. I was one of them. I have to say it felt good. I took the whole experience very seriously. It was now time to find out where we would be stationed. As we all stood together, one by one the sergeant read names off and where each would be going.

The sergeant said, "Keyes, West Pac Ground Forces." That meant Vietnam. We all received a thirty day leave. After that we were to return and attend what he called ITR. To this day I'm not sure what the initials stand for. I only knew it had to do with advance training. There we would learn how to use things like machine guns and grenades.

Home leave went by fast. I saw Mary and some of my friends and family. Mary's family threw me a birthday party. I had never had a birthday party before. Then it was time to go back. All was fine until I was back on the plane and in the air. All of sudden out of nowhere I was hit by the deepest feeling of loneliness I had ever felt in my life.

The training went well. I was made an Acting Platoon Sergeant. Again things went well as far as handling the other men. I was told I'd make a good leader. Not thinking much of the compliment, it was nice to hear though.

We were in what is called a fox hole all night as part of the training. A fox hole is a hole you dig in the ground deep enough for you and possibly another to sit in as protection while looking out for the enemy. As the night went by, questions about this war began racing through my mind. Thoughts like taking a life and losing my life. What was this war really all about in the first place? The more I thought about it the more troubled I felt. I don't know if it was a case of "You picked a fine time to think about this," or a case of "Better late than never."

After that part of the training, I started asking some of the other men why they were going. One guy said his dad fought in a war. Another said, "What would people think if I don't go." I remember thinking after that comment, "What would people think if you came back in a body bag?" I was at a loss as to what to do. I decided to talk with the officer who was in charge of our training.

I told him how I didn't understand this war and that if I was going to take a life or lose my life, it was important for me to believe in what I was about to do. Then the officer said something that struck a nerve. He said that he understood, and went on to say, "If I were you, I would go anyway." I thought to myself, that's it! He is not me, nor am I him. He isn't concerned about how I feel. His job is to get me over there. The decision came down to will things be based on what others want me to do no matter the consequences or what is best for me at this particular crossroad. I became more determined not to go.

Still troubled and not sure what to do, I decided to talk with the chaplain. He understood how I felt. When asked if he would go, without any hesitation he said, he would not go. That was all I needed to hear. My mind was made up. I had to get out of there, but how? That was the all-important question. So many things flooded my mind. I didn't want to be seen as weak or a coward. I cared about what the public thought. I cared about what my family and friends would think. I was tired of being a failure.

When it came to this particular war, I had become a conscientious-objector. I was too afraid to tell anyone that. Who would believe it and how could I prove it? If absolutely necessary, one should fight for their country. It is also vital that a person believe in what they're fighting for. When it comes to taking a life or giving my life, I must be the one to make that final decision. As bad as war is, the only just wars that I can think of is World War II, when Pearl Harbor was bombed, and the war after the 9/11 attack on the World Trade Center and the Pentagon.

So there I was, 19, feeling afraid, trapped, desperate, feeling like there was no one to talk to and having only a couple of weeks at the most to do something. All of it left me with a horrible feeling.

Early on I had heard that the one way you could get out was to be gay. I ran into another recruit that wanted out. We put a plan together and convinced the military that we were both gay. I still feel deep embarrassment and shame about what I did. Putting this out there into the light is the beginning of freeing me from this burden I've been living with.

We both ended up getting an undesirable discharge. More importantly and painful than the discharge, which was bad enough, was that this was a huge failure for that little kid in me that got some sense of self-worth from watching those war movies. This was supposed to be my chance to save the good guys. My sense of failure and sadness were so profound I suppressed that I was betraying something important to me—after all, suppressing things was something I did so well.

Little did I know that there would be no escape from being at war. While not manifesting at this point in my life, the warring factions within me were becoming established. The pain I was working to suppress from the childhood abuse was pulling me relentlessly toward the quicksand even as I struggled to find a purpose that I somehow trusted would give me the sense of worthiness I so desperately craved.

I was transferred to a special barracks (living quarters) where there were other servicemen awaiting discharges for one reason or another. None of them seemed to be getting an honorable discharge. At one point the sergeant in charge gathered us all together outside to let us know that we would all amount to nothing in life. You would have thought he would have given us encouragement instead. Looking back at the nature of the military, I understand his and their position. After all, this was the Marine Corps.

After those demoralizing comments he went back into the building. I spoke up and let the men know that our lives would be what we made them in spite of what the sergeant just said. A few more days went by, and then that same sergeant came to get me for a phone call. Who could be calling me?

When I got to the phone, on the other end was the voice of one of my siblings. She said she heard how I was getting out and that mom was crying. She went on to say I couldn't stay at home and that I should not consider myself as her brother anymore. I didn't say much; I was very hurt. It appears someone in the military called my family.

I ended up staying with my girlfriend Mary and her family for a while. A few years went by and I got the opportunity to complete my GED. Because I had finished 11th grade while in regular school, I automatically received a high school diploma, too. Getting that diploma gave my fragile sense of self-worth an unexpected boost.

More Defining Moments

I found a job working at a home for children. The management didn't seem to care for the kids, and money appeared to be the main reason for having the facility. I found myself thinking about the kids' situation day and night. My attachment to them was cemented during the Christmas holidays. I came in to work over the holidays. Some of the kids went home for the holidays, but the kids whose families didn't want them were still there. One of the kids said to me, "We know that you care because you're here with us." I made a vow to myself that I would never leave them.

Any suggestions that I made to management that I felt could improve the quality of the kids' lives seemed to fall on deaf ears. That was my first insight in understanding where the murderers, thieves, and prostitutes—the so-called misfits of society—came from. Over time, worrying about them started wearing me down. I had made that vow to never leave them.

The turning point came suddenly. I was working one day and my thoughts of not being able to help them consumed me. I reached a breaking point and just couldn't take any more. I ended up walking off the job in tears and never went back.

To truly help children, I needed more power and that meant lots of money. Where would I get it? Music made the most sense. My whole life changed drastically in those moments. The purpose for my life was realized. Going through life whichever way the wind blew me was over. Feeling like a failure because I'd made a vow to those kids and then broke it, I decided then and there to help the many kids out in the world who were being mistreated. I finally had a mission, a purpose for my life. I walked, talked, ate, and slept nothing but music, music, and music. I started taking life very seriously. I had unexpectedly found a true purpose for living.

The core of my new group was me and two members of the original singing group from high school, Clancy and Bill. Those two members became the lead singers and, along with a fourth vocalist, I took my place in the background doing harmony. That summer we took two songs that Bill wrote, pooled what little money we had together, and went into a local recording studio to cut a demo record.

This was our first experience at recording and also the first time singing with a three-piece band—drums, bass guitar, and conga—put together for the occasion. The studio time was about

$25 an hour. We ended up making a very good single recording. Back in those days singles were made on a vinyl disc called a 45. A main song was recorded on one side, called the A side, and a second song, usually thought to be less significant, was recorded on the second or B side.

A couple of months later, through a friend, we were introduced to someone who knew the music business very well. He listened to our demo, talked to a distributor, and then told us to put together four sets of music, each set consisting of 45 minutes' worth of music to perform at local bars. This wasn't what I wanted to hear. I wanted to make big money right away on a record deal. The manager said we needed to perform more and get known. Once we drew a good following, we could cut a record for release. If enough local fans bought the record, it could propel us to a national level. So we had a plan. As leader of the group, it fell on my shoulders to keep the band together, put together the four sets, and make sure we learned them.

The manager made me aware of the importance of listening. He told us, "Successful groups listen to who's in charge." He said the downfall of most male groups was drugs and women. He said that if you start messing with women it could upset their men. The men needed to like our band, too. He also explained the importance of performing cover tunes (other popular artists' songs) that are familiar to our audiences until we got better known. It all made sense to me.

The part regarding other artist songs bothered Bill. As a songwriter, he wanted to do originals and artist songs that had radical messages. Although hesitant, I initially went along with Bill because of our long-standing friendship and his overall importance to the group as a songwriter and vocalist. Was this to become my first serious test as a leader? When we did our first full performance at a bar filled with young people who just wanted to party and dance, some of them ended up walking out on us when we did the radical songs. My goal to help children was being jeopardized.

When it came time to meet with the manager, which I did on a weekly basis, I explained what happened on our first job. He again explained the importance of doing the right songs at the right time. I went back to the group and shared that information with them. Bill remained rebellious. He thought we shouldn't sell out. "Sell out" was a very strong term. I understood where Bill was coming from but thought we should listen to someone who knew the business. In other words, we should play cards until we were in a position to deal. As the leader, I was confronted with a very important decision. Should I risk following someone I didn't know well, that is the manager, and be seen as a sellout by the band members? Especially by Bill, who was more to me than just a member of the group? When I had no place to stay, it was Bill and his family who invited me into their family. They never once made me feel unwelcome.

The decision was made. We would follow the manager's knowledgeable advice and not do songs that were controversial. In anger and defiance, Bill persuaded Clancy, our best lead singer, not to attend rehearsals. After talking with both of them and getting nowhere, I decided to move on without them. It was a very painful decision, but my commitment to helping kids was far more important. Both were replaced with satisfactory singers. When Mom put me out of the house, I learned that love and life are two different things. Here I was putting two core people who meant a lot to the group and to me personally out of the group. It was painful.

With the new group, our vocal harmonies were not quite as good as before but they were good enough and we were pretty evenly skilled. Now all singers could do lead vocal work, including me. This gave us more variety as a public appearance group. We ended up becoming one of the top show groups in the state. We added nonstop choreography. After the first few songs, we were soaked with sweat. We went from being the band that was walked out on to the band that people could not get in to see because of the crowds. We always critiqued our performances and worked hard at practices to correct what we did wrong. And that's what separated us from most groups of that time.

Because of the manager, we got the opportunity to perform with two nationally known groups and held our own. A group called the Ides of March had a hit record out called *Vehicle*, and Edwin Starr, had a hit record called *War*. Because of the hit record they had, each member of the Ides of March netted $90 thousand in public appearances in one year. That was a lot of money back then. My dream to help children was becoming closer.

The time had come, and we were ready to record our first professional record. The manager wanted all of us to write original material for the record. While in a motel room on one of our gigs, I stayed up all night writing my first song. Called *Who Am I*, the song sums up my attempt at age 25 to understand my purpose and life's meaning (see Songs and Poems).

The manager decided to use another member's original. Once recorded, it took another year before the record was released. If we could get into the Top 10 on one of the most popular Top 40 radio stations, we would be guaranteed some big successes. We reached number 12. Our public appearances went up a few hundred dollars. The booking agents felt good about the higher money. The agent came to me one day excited about a $600 job he had gotten us for doing one 45-minute set. I admit that wasn't bad money, but because of my goal to help the children, I told him I would not be satisfied until we were making $10,000 a night. The agent called the manager and asked him, "What's wrong with Louie?"

Chapter 4

Life Starts Splintering

Leading the band was important to me. I wanted to be a good leader, and I wanted the band to be a success. I developed many leadership skills I lacked as I went along. But I was also learning that desire alone does not promise success. I only came to the understanding many years later that there are things that you cannot control, and so you need to increase your chances by optimizing what you can control. For example, you need to live a balanced life so you can lead from strength instead of weakness. You have to get proper rest, exercise, and nutrients to be at your very best. You may get away with a haphazard life style and too much pressure for a while. But not forever.

Breakdown at Age 26

For three years I put all my energy into running the group and trying to make it big so that I could help children with the money I earned. I ran a disciplined group. If you broke the rules more than once you had to go. The group's makeup changed three times or more in those three years. I was wearing down from the stress. I was not eating, exercising, or sleeping right. I was always anxious and could never sit still for long.

Odd things started happening. Signs of my mental deterioration although I didn't realize it then. We had a music van for the band, and I remember waking up early one morning, jumping into the van, and starting to drive like I had an appointment somewhere only to realize I didn't even know where I was going or why I had started driving in the first place.

On the day of my mental breakdown, I had been smoking marijuana and ended up in a bar thinking three people were there to kill me. With my mind in a total panic, I ran out of the bar and onto a city bus that happened to be right outside with its door open. Through the whole ride I kept thinking someone was going to get on the bus at each stop and try to kill me.

Once back in the hotel room where I was staying at the time, I called a friend and tried to explain what had happened. When he asked me why they were after me, I panicked even more and lost my voice. I thought he was in on it. He kept saying, "Hello? Hello?" Every time I tried to speak, nothing came out. He hung up. I called him right back and when he said, "Hello?" I still could not talk as hard as I tried.

I was on one of the top floors of the hotel. I got a piece of paper and started a fire to try and get the attention of someone walking by on the streets below. I quickly put the fire out thinking they might think I was crazy. Feeling trapped, I called down to the front desk to try and get help. When the clerk said, "Hello?" I hung up thinking he was in on it.

Not long after, there was a knock at the door and a voice said they were the police. I thought they were there to kill me. The police asked me to come along with them. I thought they were going to kill me in the hallway. When we got on the elevator, I thought they were going to kill me there. Once we got down to the lobby and the door opened, a man walked by and I thought he was there to kill me. By that time I was emotionally spent.

Once in the lobby I asked if I could call my mother. I told her I just called to say I love you and that I was sorry for all the trouble I caused her growing up. I hung up and proceeded outside to the police van with the two officers. I thought they were going to kill me in there. After that didn't happen, I thought they were going to kill me at the police station. They ended up instead taking me to the Mental Health Complex. I thought someone was going to kill me there.

After spending the weekend in the hospital and feeling obsessed with my goal of making it in music to help kids, I told the doctor I had important things I had to do. I was released Monday morning. I stopped by a restaurant to have breakfast. While sitting there waiting, I felt a calmness that was alien to me. On one level I had music on my mind and on another the fear of knowing that someone wanted to hurt me. If someone had spoken to me, I wouldn't have known how to respond. I wanted to jump up and run out of the place but I didn't.

When I saw the group members the following day at a scheduled rehearsal, I informed them about the breakdown but gave no details. I went on to say that I was leaving the group but that I would continue to work on the outside for them. I felt this was still my group. After all, I started the group from scratch, and no one was as committed or had put as much energy and time in making the group a success as I had. I didn't come this far to give up now. Not long after, though, the group fell into the hands of another member they chose to follow. For me, this was heartbreaking. Six months later the group broke up. I learned that any successful organization has to have a leader. Others can say things that sound good but in the end no one can see what you see.

My determination to make it did not falter even after the breakdown and losing the group. All along when I was in the group, people told me that I was good enough to go on my own. The only problem was that I had only known the security of a group. I didn't have the confidence to go on my own. Now I was forced to. With a few original songs I had written, some clothes, and some borrowed money for a one-way airplane ticket, I headed for New York City.

I had never been to New York City and knew no one there. I got a room at the YMCA. The next day I started off to make my dream come true. The first record company I stopped at was United Artists. They said they weren't looking for new talent at the time. I stopped off at Columbia Records and that also was a dead end. Next stop was Atlantic Records. Finally there was some hope. I was taken to a room where there was a piano. Soon another gentleman who was a piano player came in just to listen. I performed one of my original songs and they seemed to like it. I was told to come back the next day and share my remaining songs.

This was starting to look like my big break. I would never know though. I started thinking that all they wanted to do was steal my songs. I never went back. I ran out of money and ended up staying at a rescue mission that night. They directed me the next day to a place where I could eat for free. Hopeless and lost, I tried to sell my clothes to a parking attendant. When he refused to take them I threw the clothes down and told him to just keep them and then stormed off.

It was dark and getting late. Out of complete desperation and fear, I called the police. As I was explaining my situation to the officer, I heard laughter in the background and the officer on the phone with me began to laugh, too. I just knew they were all laughing at my situation and at me. I slammed the phone down and walked off.

The only thing I could think of now was to check myself into a mental institution. I found a hospital called Bellevue. They admitted me and put me on some medication. As I lay there in the dark, powerless to move, I was gripped by fear thinking that here I was in a city where I knew no one and in a hospital where anything could happen.

The next day I was given some more medication that caused a spasm in my back so that I couldn't walk straight. The nurse gave me another pill that fixed that problem. After a few days, I became very restless. I asked if I could go anywhere else. They suggested another mental illness facility called Staten Island, but later a nurse I asked about the place told me I didn't want to go there.

After a few more restless days, I said I wanted to go to the Staten Island facility. Unlike Bellevue, I was put in a large room with about twenty-five other men. Everybody slept on army cots side by side. People's clothing was stolen. Someone's bed was set on fire. It was truly a crazy place. One day when I was at the end of the line waiting to eat, a younger patient started at the front and systematically went down the line slapping everyone. When he got to me our eyes met; the guy skipped over me.

After about a month, friends in Chicago put together the money so I could catch a plane back. I went straight to my dad's house. He had been ill from a heart attack.

I prayed that he was all right. When I got to his house, Dad was resting in bed. He had no idea what had happened to me. Dad asked me what I was going to do with my life. I had no idea. I had no money. I had nowhere to stay. I checked myself back into a mental institution.

After three months, I was encouraged to try and find a job, so I went out looking during the day. I successfully applied at a foundry. I had never worked in a foundry before. They gave me a tour and showed me where I would be working. The place looked like something you'd see in a movie representing hell. What looked like fog was really black soot from the fiery furnaces and hot molten metal that was being carried around in these huge containers on a trolley line throughout the plant. The molten metal sometimes spilled out onto the ground and hot sparks flew everywhere. Some spilled near me and I jumped. The nearby workers started laughing.

After the tour, I stepped back outside into the sunlight and fresh air. Even just after a short tour, my nose was full of soot. What would eight hours or more be like under those conditions? The next day I found out. My job was to load up a wheelbarrow full of metal, walk it over to a hole in the floor, and dump it. This was to be done nonstop until break time. It wasn't long before I was exhausted and in pain. During the break, I went into the locker room to eat. The room was full of that cloudy soot. That was it. Discouraged and defeated, I walked off the job.

Still determined to find work, I saw a well-known department store across the street. I applied and got that job, too. Not long after I was able to check out of the hospital and get a room at a friend's relative's house. After working in the warehouse for a few weeks, I was promoted to installer of washers and dryers in customers' homes. Not only did I get my own van, I could also take it home with me.

In 1975, I had been working for almost two years. It was the longest I had ever worked any job. The economy started going downhill, and I was part of what was called "a reduction in force." Simply put, I no longer had a job.

The loss of that job put a lot of stress on me, as it would anyone. I couldn't find any job that paid the same or close. I couldn't pay my rent and was evicted. Destitute, stressed out, and feeling lost, I decided to go back to the mental hospital. I was shocked when the intake doctor said he wasn't going to allow me in. With my back to the wall, I said if I was not allowed in, I was going to go outside, get my jack out of my car, and start breaking windows.

He still refused. I got up, went outside, and got my jack out of the trunk of my car. I walked over to a huge plate glass window and made sure no one was sitting by it, then I threw the jack as hard as I could. The window vibrated but didn't break. I picked up the jack and tried again. The same thing happened. This time I grabbed the jack and headed for the door to the hospital. As I opened the door to enter, that intake doctor stepped through the second door and said, "Okay! Okay! I'll admit you."

I went in and sat down in the same chair feeling great relief. He sat down in front of me and said, "I'm still not going to admit you." I pulled my arm back with a clenched fist like I was going to hit him even though I knew that I wasn't. As I came forward with my clenched fist, he covered himself with both arms. At that same moment, a sheriff walked into the office. The doctor must have called him while I was out in the parking lot. I said, "I didn't hit him," and walked out.

I got in my car and sped off like I had lost my mind. I no longer wanted to live. Life was too painful. I calmed down as I thought about ways to end my life. I continued driving. I remembered this mental hospital I had seen as I was driving through a small town one day, and it wasn't far away. I decided to go there and see if they would admit me. If they did take me in, I would think of that as a good sign; if not, I would find something I could ram my car into that would kill me and not hurt anyone else. The doctor at the small hospital admitted me.

At first I didn't have much to say to anyone, but after two weeks I started talking. One day one of the counselors I felt comfortable with took me to his office to talk. As people walked by his open door, I explained how the colors they were wearing affected my thinking. I talked to him like I'd talk to a trusted friend. Suddenly he became angry and said, "Stop it." He thought I was making it up to manipulate him. I felt incredibly hurt and confused. A day or so later I was in a psychologist's office and he showed me a book called *Games People Play*. I'm not sure if he was trying to say something about my encounter with the counselor or not. Seeing that book cover made it even more unlikely that I would mention my experiences with colors.

Two weeks later I was discharged. I was able to get a room in the area through social services. I had rested just enough to continue on with my life.

It was not unusual for me to not contact family members for months at a time. Since I hadn't talked to anyone for a while, I called home and found out they had buried Dad the day before I was discharged. They had tried to find me. They had even broadcast their search on a local radio station. I didn't feel much when told of Dad's death. He died of a heart attack. I only started grieving his death years later in a dream.

In the dream, I was running down the middle of a street trying to get away. Everyone was chasing me and trying to control me. I was having none of it. Soon I saw a lady in a white dress standing calmly by the side of the road near a house. I ran right past her to the back of the house. I ran up some stairs into this unfamiliar house. As I got halfway up, somehow I knew my father was in that house dying. I stopped and tremendous sadness welled up inside. I felt like my heart was about to burst with grief. I woke up.

The Force

After the breakdown and first hospital stay, I was no longer the same person. My awareness and sensitivity level greatly increased. A general sense of being afraid was taking over my days. I think because I was so preoccupied with my music career and because it happened so gradually and subtly, I didn't recognize that I was becoming more and more fearful. After the New York experience, I struggled desperately to figure out where I belonged. I felt deeply lost and alone. My sense of purpose had all but gone. It truly felt like death. As a relentless search to find new purpose and meaning began, normal everyday things started taking on heightened and odd meanings. I was totally unaware that I was suffering from a mental illness that was getting progressively worse. I eventually called what was happening to me the "Force" because I started feeling compelled to do things I didn't want to do. It got to the point where I could no longer discern my thoughts from truth. If I thought it, it was real. In the movie *Star Wars*, the Force was seen as good. It was the opposite for me.

About nine months after the first breakdown, I was in a large department store at a mall shopping when all of a sudden I had a panic attack. It seemed as though everyone in the store was trying to control me just like in that dream I had about my dad dying in that unfamiliar house. The people in the store trying to control me included the store clerks and other shoppers; old people, young people, and even little children were in on it. Everyone in that store was out to get me in some way.

I rushed to the east exit as fast as I could. When I got outside I came to a dead stop. I peered out into the parking lot unsure of what to do next. I pretended I was looking for my car. Feeling helpless and trapped, I started looking at one of the bright yellow lines that the cars parked between. My thoughts flashed back to what a gentleman had said to me years earlier. He told me I had to walk a straight line. It had bothered me that I didn't understand what he meant.

As inconspicuously as I could, I walked out to that yellow line still pretending I was looking for my car and just stood on it. In that moment I wanted so badly to have it together just like the people around me. Standing on that line somehow gave me a little break from the terror I was feeling. I slowly started walking down the line still pretending I was looking for my car. When I came to the end of that line, I just stood there not knowing what to do next. I knew I couldn't stand there forever. Someone might get suspicious and think I was up to no good.

After standing on that yellow line for what seemed like forever, I finally gathered up all the emotional courage and physical strength I had left and forced myself off the line. I went to my car and drove off feeling deep relief. I think this helped cement some of the odd relationships I began seeing between colors and my feelings.

Keyes County

I tried to work but my lack of stability kept getting in the way. Time and time again I found a job, overreacted to something someone said or did, and quit. In some cases I walked off in the middle of a job without saying a word to anyone because I was bored or just didn't like the job. In one particular year I worked twelve different jobs. I moved from one town to another looking for that perfect job and that perfect town where I would be accepted and could finally call home. I would move into a town, get free help through social services, drop the help once I found a job, and then lose the job and move again. I became so desperate that one day as I was looking at a map I saw on it a county with my last name. I became excited thinking that this had to be that special place that I had been searching for. This would be the town where I could find acceptance and rest. I could call the town with my name my home.

I jumped on a Greyhound bus and off I went. I had enough money to spend one night in a hotel. Again I was counting on social services to help me. The bus got into town early evening. My anticipation was high. Social services was right across the street from the bus depot but was closed for the day. I got a room and went the very next day to social services and they got me a room. Things were falling into place.

At first the landlord seemed nice enough. You had to share a restroom with other roomers in the building. Nothing was said about a shower. I discovered that there was one on the floor below, so I went down and took a shower. When the landlord found out, he was furious and told me that I had to leave. Feeling hurt and confused, I grabbed my few belongings and left, not sure what to do next.

One block down across the street, I saw a sign in the window of a hardware store. It was advertising a room for rent. I went in, met the owner, and got the room, which was upstairs from the store. The owner was very nice. And the room had a shower in it. I had some house painting experience and ended up doing some work for the owner.

One day as I was walking around town, I saw the strangest thing. It was a horse hooked up to a black carriage and the people getting out of it had on strange clothes that were mostly black.

The women had on bonnets and long dresses. Two little kids were dressed in the same style of clothing, like little adults. It was the neatest thing to see. Later on I found out they were called Amish.

Eventually as time went by, I saved up enough money to buy a nice used car. I saw the Amish a few more times in town. I also found out they were farmers and lived out on the west side of town. One day I decided to go and look for these neat looking people. As I was driving around in the country, I noticed a man with Amish-style clothing out by the road that led to a farmhouse. I stopped, got out of the car, walked up to the young looking man, and introduced myself. To my amazement, when the man introduced himself, he said, "My name is Louie, too." Now what was the chance of that? The first Amish man I met had the same name as me!

One of the spellbinding ways in which the Force affected me more and more was through colors. I'm not sure but it might be so that one of the reasons the Amish people seemed safe to me was because their clothing had no color to mix me up. When driving or walking, colors sometimes made it difficult if not impossible for me to get to a particular destination. For instance, suppose I was driving along and saw a red car. If the car was coming towards me or moving in the same direction or parked, each situation affected me differently. If a red car was parked, I might wonder if I was supposed to stop, so I would immediately start an intense search scanning the area for what the Force wanted me to do. Sometimes I pulled over, parked the car, and saw someone walk out of a building. So then I might wonder if the Force wanted me to go into the building where another message might be waiting.

If I went in and saw some people talking, I tried to get as close to them as possible without making it obvious so I could listen for a message coming through them to me from the Force. I looked at their clothing to see if they reminded me of another person or place, anything. If no one was around, I looked for pictures on the wall to see what secrets they might hold. I could find a meaning or message in most anything. My stress level affected how much influence the Force had on me at any given time. The more stress, the more active the Force became.

If I decided not to stop after seeing the parked red car, my odd thinking continued. "Maybe the Force is telling me that I forgot to do something. I didn't cook anything when I was at home so I couldn't have left the stove or oven on. I'm sure I locked the door when I left the house."

I might try to put the Force out of my mind but then another red car crossed the intersection in front of me. This time because the red car was two tones, the second color green, I took it to mean the Force wanted me to go in another direction. I figured it wanted me to see something. What that something was I had no way of knowing so I kept alert for anything and everything. I searched and searched for a sign, studying people's clothing, faces, anything that might tell me what to do next. I looked at houses, their colors, shapes and sizes, and animals if any were around.

Tired and frustrated, I frantically looked for whatever the Force was trying to tell me. Then yet another red car caught my attention, and I took that to mean I should pull over and park again. I pulled over and parked and waited for the Force to tell me what to do or not to do, where to go or not to go. I was afraid to go on without a sign from the Force.

Finally a blue and green car came by, and I took that to mean I should start driving again. Feeling mentally and emotionally exhausted by now, I started the car and started driving aimlessly in a daze. A brown and tan car goes by and I start following it. A silver car goes by and I start following it. Now I notice a parked red car so I turn at the next intersection since now a red car means I should switch directions. As I turn I see another car with red in it so I turn again and see a person walking wearing all blue so I look up at the blue sky to see if some kind of message is up there. I continue on and on, turning again and again, parking and driving, trying to follow the directions of the Force. Finally, I'm back home. When morning comes, the Force is waiting.

One day I was in my apartment feeling very upset about an incident that took place in a local bar. I decided I would go back and give that person a piece of my mind. Upon leaving the apartment, I opened the door that led outside and noticed a cricket in the corner just behind the door. I was feeling a lot of anger and as I looked hard at the cricket, it started jumping up and down in a frantic way. I believed the Force was coming through that cricket's frantic behavior to warn me not to return to that bar. I went back upstairs to my apartment and looked out the window and saw some ducks landing in a pond. I looked at the clock and it was around noon, so the Force was telling me through the ducks that it was time to eat.

As the months passed, my paranoia became more and more deeply rooted in my personality. I thought the radio and TV were giving me messages. I would listen to complete strangers in a grocery store and believe that they were giving me secret messages. I believed that things were being put into my food to hurt me. If I went into a personnel office looking for work and the phone rang, I thought it was someone telling the personnel receptionist that they should not give me a job.

Deeper Hell

Ten years had passed since the first breakdown and things started to get even worse. Tired and worn out, disillusioned and desperate from the pressures of listening and doing what the Force wanted me to do, my strange thinking escalated. My thoughts started to become homicidal.

I started thinking that the reason things weren't going right for me was because the Force wanted me to kill people. The thought frightened me but over time the homicidal thoughts became stronger and more pronounced. The messages were now about who to kill, how to kill, and when to kill. I eventually committed several homicides.

As bizarre as my thinking was during the crimes, it still made sense to me at the time. I know how strange that sounds to someone who has not experienced paranoid thinking or delusions. The delusional thinking needed to make a kind of sense or I needed to make a kind of sense out of the thoughts or they could not have taken hold the way they did. I really do not want to talk about it because I have deep shame, sorrow, and guilt about what I did. I have decided that it's important no matter how I feel to give one or two samples of my thinking during this period of my life when the mental illness was strongest.

For example, I was living in Beloit and had landed a job painting the outside of a house for two very nice elderly ladies. One day I visited Cascade, a town about 200 miles away where I had lived one year. While visiting I ran into a gentleman who was senior manager of the hotel I was staying in. He and his family had treated me well when I lived there before. In conversation I found out that the night manager was giving the senior manager a hard time and wanted his position. I didn't like it that the night manager was giving someone who had been nice to me a hard time, but it was only a passing thought at the time.

I returned to Beloit and one evening after a day of painting, the two ladies pulled up into the driveway. They had been shopping. While helping them take their groceries into the house, one of them made a comment to the other about hurrying up or they would be late.

I immediately started thinking about the senior manager of the hotel in Cascade. Were the comments made by the two elderly ladies about being late a secret message from the Force? Was the senior manager in danger from the night manager who wanted his job? Was the Force trying to tell me that getting back there as soon as possible was imperative? That I needed to hurry or I would be too late to save him?

I quickly made up a story that something had come up and I had to go out of town for a few days. I asked the two elderly ladies if they could advance me some money to make the trip and told them the house would get finished as soon as I got back. Their willingness to lend me the money and their understanding made me know my thinking was on the right track.

Upon arrival I checked into the hotel. Both the senior manager and the night manager were there. My sensitivity was on high alert for signs from the Force about what to do next. I had a strong sense that the night manager had to be killed, but it didn't make sense that someone needed to die over a hotel job. The next day while I was visiting friends, I heard that someone had killed his girlfriend some years back and never been caught. I don't recall now if I heard it in conversation or while reading the paper or listening to the radio. "It must be this night manager who killed his girlfriend," I thought. "That's why he must die." Now I needed messages from the Force telling me how, when, and where.

The night manager lived by himself in a two bedroom apartment. After getting to know him through small talk, I asked him if I could move in until I was able to find a job and get my own place. He agreed. The how was answered soon. First the Force allowed me to purchase a gun at a store. The fact that I could buy the gun made it obvious to me that the gun was part of the Force's plan. Then while out at a restaurant, I overheard people talking about having some kind of car trouble. I took this as another hidden message from the Force. I was to pretend I had car trouble.

The next message I was looking for from the Force was when and where. The night manager had taken me to a job interview and we traveled a less used road to get there. A less used road was just what I needed. Clearly another message. To pull this off without getting caught, I needed to arrange an opportunity late at night and during the week when most people are home and asleep. Was that the Force telling me? Or was that one of those odd moments of clarity that I had on my own? I don't know any more. I called him about 1:00 A.M. and told him that my car had broken down out on that lonely road. If he refused to come help me, it would be a message from the Force that he was to be spared, but he agreed. I must be reading the messages correctly. He came to help me, and I killed him.

This second example of delusional thinking made even more sense to me at the time. I knew a lady name Connie for a bit before I met Jed. He was a quiet man, and I didn't know him well. Jed and Connie were engaged to be married after a very short relationship. One weekend when I was in the process of moving, I needed a place to stay and Jed agreed to accommodate me.

Shortly after I arrived at Jed's house, I realized that he was in a bad space. Connie had called off the engagement. Jed started talking about her in a berating way; it was Connie this and Connie that. This went on for quite some time. I said gently, "Face it, Jed, you're hurt." Jed flew into a rage and started yelling at me about how I didn't know anything and accused me and Connie with having something going on ourselves. He stood with his face inches from mine with his face showing the strain and veins popping out on his neck.

After he calmed down, we talked a little and went to bed. The very next morning he asked me to leave. I was concerned about the level of his anger so I decided to share my concerns with a couple who knew him hoping they would look in on him. They had this odd antique-looking camera that would later play a part in my delusion. I also thought it best to let Connie know how angry and upset Jed was.

I lived and worked about three hours away from the town where Connie and Jed lived. I had a nice job singing karaoke as background music at a local supper club. Things were going well in my new place. To supplement my income, I stopped by a real-estate office hoping I could find some side work like painting. In the office was this same antique-like camera I saw at Jed's friends' home.

Unhappily, a month later, my boss told me that they would have to let me go in a week because of lack of business. It was a big disappointment. The stress was building. I knew the Force was responsible for the job loss. It was letting me know that I had an assignment to kill someone.

I moved into an inexpensive motel. I started thinking about Charlie, someone I had met who lived above his elderly landlord about 10 miles away in the country. Charlie must be the target I thought. I had a small pistol in my pocket, but I truly did not want to hurt this person. Also, I knew he had a rifle.

I got to Charlie's place and as we sat talking, I started thinking about that little pistol and what if it didn't work and what if he got ahold of that rifle. He said that the landlord was out of town for a few days. I decided I could wait another day and left.

Back in the town where I was living, I stopped downtown to pick up some lay-away items. When I stepped back outside, I was watching all the people when I suddenly felt that the Force wanted me to kill everybody I saw. This had never happened before. That was the first time that I wondered if something was wrong with me. I had killed several people already and there I was only then wondering if something might be wrong with me! I had been so sure at the time that I was doing what needed to be done for the good of someone else.

I headed back to the motel feeling very nervous. They had a small restaurant and I decided to get some coffee hoping the Force could direct me in what to do. As I sat, I listened to the conversations of other customers looking for one that was telling me what I was supposed to do. I heard nothing helpful. I looked at the pictures on the wall hoping to find something that made sense. Then I spotted a calendar hanging high on the wall with a picture of a little girl on her knees praying. The girl looked exactly like Connie! The large heading on the calendar said Something Something Funeral Home. I thought, "Oh my God! Jed is going to kill Connie!" The camera in the real estate office that looked just like the one in Jed's friends' home meant Jed was also part of the Force's secret message. It all made perfect sense now. The Force didn't want me to kill the guy in the country. The Force wanted me to kill Jed.

I gassed up the car and started the three hour trip to stop Jed. Even though I didn't want to hurt him, I couldn't let him kill Connie. I still wanted more assurance that what I was about to do was right. I stopped at several stores hoping to see more messages confirming the assignment. I really hoped I was reading the messages wrong despite the evidence. Unhappily, I knew that I was right.

I drove to a store a few blocks from Jed's house where he and I had shopped together. I was hoping for a message letting me know what to do. There was none. I pulled up in front of Jed's house knowing that he got off late, but hoping he wouldn't come home at all. That would be a message. Soon Jed pulled up. I was hoping he wouldn't let me in the house. That would be a message. When I asked to come in, he kind of reluctantly said, "Yes." The house was quite a mess. On the table was a revolver. It was clear to me in that split second that he was going to kill Connie and that was why the Force had given me the assignment to kill him.

Sharing all this from a position of recovery is very difficult. I feel deep shame and pain. I just want to lie down and never get up again. I felt tremendous anguish in taking each life. I spent countless sleepless nights praying for answers and experiencing the torturous twisting need to confide in someone but too much fear to countermand the Force. I thought everyone knew what I was doing, but the Force didn't want me talking to anyone about it.

My body ached with fear. I thought, "How would people treat me? What would they do if they knew? They might hurt me; they won't like me; they might lock me up; I can't tell them; they know; maybe they don't know; I have to do what I'm doing but I really don't want to hurt anyone; God says, thou shall not kill, but who will protect the good people? Why do I have to do it? Maybe I'm the only one who can. I want to tell someone. God, please, if you're out there, help me. Am I doing the right thing? Thou shall not kill."

Before I committed the final homicide, I was driving through a little town and saw a mental health sign on a building. The Force had already picked out a victim that I didn't want to hurt. I decided to stop in the mental health agency. An intake worker came and greeted me. As we were talking I tried to tell him what was happening. I said, "What if I told you I thought I was supposed to kill somebody?" He quickly said in a very stern way, "I'd take you upstairs and lock you right up!" An image flashed in my mind of my dad yelling, "Shut up!" while he was beating me as a child. I knew this was the Force's way of telling me not to talk about it, so I left. The Force required fear and secrecy and obedience. I didn't dare talk about the Force or I would be punished in some way.

It Ends

As the two detectives approached, I thought they just wanted to talk and ask more questions about the murder that had taken place a few days ago. But they drew their guns and said, "You're under arrest for the murder of Jed Smith." I felt numb and indifferent as they walked me to the awaiting police car in handcuffs.

I denied killing Jed even though I thought the police knew about my secret mission even without me telling them about it. Not talking made me feel special and powerful. At the same time, not talking also made me feel very lonely. The detectives asked me if I wanted a lawyer, and I said, "No." I thought they would soon let me go. After all, why would they keep someone they knew was on his secret mission? Then the detectives asked me if I would be willing to take a lie detector test, and I said, "Sure." On the one hand my parents basically raised me up to tell the truth and that lying was wrong. I knew if the machine really worked the tester would know I was lying. But on the other hand, my secret thoughts knew that the tester would say that I passed so I could continue my missions. I gave the police my full cooperation with the exception of admitting to the crimes I had committed. In my secret thoughts, I knew they knew what I was doing and just needed a seemingly legitimate way to let me go. I couldn't tell them what I'd done or about my missions because then they couldn't find a way to let me go. It was like the book cover for *The Games People Play.*

The gentleman giving the lie detector test was very polite and friendly, which made me feel even more confident that I would soon be on my way. He was clearly part of the Force's plan. After taking the lie detector test, I sat with the detectives waiting for the results and talking about my goals regarding music and making money to help children. Everyone was treating me so nice.

Soon the polite tester returned with the test results. He pulled up a chair, sat right in front of me, and said in a very serious jarring way, "You are lying." I sat there speechless and stunned. I thought to myself, "This is not the way it's supposed to happen." I admitted to the homicide.

On the way back to the jail, I still thought they were going to let me go. I couldn't figure out, though, how they were going to manage it. I racked my mind wondering what I should do next. I knew that how I behaved and what I said would make a difference so the Force could arrange for me to go on with my missions. When we got back to the jail, the detectives started questioning me again. They started asking me about a different homicide. Again I resisted telling them, but soon, in deep despair, I confessed to that one also.

They asked me again if I wanted an attorney. I said, "Yes." I still thought we were just going through some required steps so they could somehow let me go. We all knew what was really going on and the importance of my mission. Maybe saying no to the lawyer before had been the wrong answer for the plan. Maybe saying yes now would make it work.

In the cell bunk that night, the emotional pain was far too great to bear. Confused and in utter despair, tears streaming down my face, I kept hitting the cell wall with my fists and asking why was this happening? Again in my mind, I was only trying to play what I thought was my part in this confusing game. I sincerely believed I had finally found my purpose in life as painful as it was. I thought I finally mattered. Late into the night I kept crying out to God, "Please God, if you're out there and really care, don't let me wake up and see another day. Please God, kill me, please." Drenched in tears, over and over I kept repeating that prayer. I stayed up all night making a plan about what to say to the lawyer. I figured he would know that I was lying, but if it was a good lie, it would give them the excuse they needed to let me go. Not being able to sleep, I spent the remainder of the night making a plan.

When my attorney came in the next morning, we met in a little room and he introduced himself and started asking me questions. I put my plan into action but after only two sentences came out my mouth, unimpressed, he stopped me dead in my tracks. He did it without even looking at me as he continued to write things down. It was as though he knew instantly that I was not being truthful. Again the tears came. All that work I put in during the night dreaming up the perfect lie to help them let me go so I could continue my missions was wasted.

Now I will be seen as this terrible uncaring person who thought only of himself. Maybe I wasn't as caring as I thought I was and just maybe they were still going to somehow let me go. I wished I could be waking up from a bad dream.

The media was relentless. Hour after hour, day after day, it was Louie Keyes this and Louie Keyes that. The shame and embarrassment I felt was overwhelming. I started thinking about the victims and the tremendous grief and anger their loved ones, friends, and neighbors were feeling and also those who cared for me. All that pain caused by me thinking I was doing the right thing, thinking this would make me a valued member of society.

Red Tie Incident

At one of the initial court hearings, one of my two public defenders wore a red tie. That screaming red tie immediately attracted my attention. The Force's message was as clear as day. Red meant stop. Because the tie was around his neck, the Force was telling me I should not speak. I clenched my teeth and pressed my lips together as tightly as I could. I was paralyzed with fear. What should I do if my attorneys or the judge asked me a question? This was a hearing and someone was sure to ask me a question. How would it look if I refused to talk? Please! Don't ask me any questions! I fought back the tears and concentrated on hoping they would not call me to the stand. Maybe I could get away with just a nod. If my attorney asked me something, maybe I could give just a very short answer. I put the plan into effect. I only nodded and said, "Uh uh," to any question. It was a great relief when that hearing ended. At some time much later I told my attorney about this, and he later referred to it as "the red tie incident."

Denial

I still identified with and trusted the police more than my attorneys. After all, the police were the good guys, and I was helping them by getting rid of the so-called bad guys, which made me a good guy, too. We were on the same side. When my attorneys talked to me face to face, I trusted them, but as soon as they left my thinking changed, my trust quickly evaporated, and I became suspicious. I started thinking they were working with the district attorney against me.

Because of my distrust for my attorneys and trust for the police, my attorneys could not defend me, so I was sent down to the hospital for a competency evaluation. While at the hospital, I was always trying to be helpful to those around me and when the doctor asked me questions related to competency, I always knew the answers.

One time when I got back from the hospital and was feeling pretty good, I entered the cell and it was as if the illness was crouched in the corner waiting for me. Within minutes the paranoia consumed me again. My emotions kept rapidly cycling from fear to anger, then to sadness, then laughter, and back to fear again, all within seconds. I had never experienced that before. After my arrest, an officer had asked me if I thought I was mentally ill. I said I just had problems like everyone else. After this experience in my cell I started thinking that maybe something really *was* wrong with me.

It was very difficult coming to the realization that I was mentally ill. I was in total denial. There was no way that I could possibly be ill! I spent most of my life working on becoming an accepted and valued member of society.

In trying to decide in my own mind if I should just go to prison or pursue an insanity plea, a loved one made this caring comment after she realized how ill I was. She said, "Louie, you don't know what it's like to be mentally healthy." My desire to be okay, just to be normal, was deeply entrenched. I remember breaking down in tears several times when I finally realized that not only was I ill, there would be no quick fix.

Although I had never heard voices before, I remember while in the cell one day I heard a voice as clear as day say "Louie." I recognized the person saying it instantly. It was a guy named Ron who used to be a member of my vocal group, and I hadn't seen him in years. I thought the guards had piped his voice in the cell some kind of way and were messing with me.

After the competency evaluations and court hearings, I was sentenced to a mental hospital and placed in maximum security. Even then, I still hadn't fully accepted the fact that I was ill.

Chapter 5

Recovery

On maximum security, the doctor soon put me on medication after I told staff about some violent thinking I was having towards two peers that I felt were trouble. I was very open and honest about my thoughts and told them that I would not follow through with any of my thoughts. Because I was new and they didn't know me, they couldn't take the chance. I felt betrayed when they moved me to an even more secure unit. The doctor said if I didn't take medication, the hospital would get a court order. That meant they could physically force it on me. I took the medication. What else could I do?

I went from being energetic to wanting to sleep all the time. I could sleep straight through the night, wake up, and feel like I had never been to sleep. After eight months of this I asked the doctor if he would take me off, and he said, "So you want to rough it?" I said, "Yes I want to rough it." And let me tell you, it was rough!

My energy and alertness soon returned. I knew that if I was going to remain medication-free, I had to find my way out of this hellish maze of confusion I was trapped in. All I had at that time was bulldog determination. I thought to myself, "I wasn't born crazy, so there has to be a way to figure this out."

It's interesting to me that an important part of my recovery turned out to be thinking about and facing the reality of my past, the world and people around me, my choices, and my actions. Using logic was very important and logic was something I didn't have as much access to when I was medicated. Equally important, if not more, turned out to be finding the courage to feel my emotions. I had to relive and experience the full brunt of my deepest fears, hurts, shame, and anger without acting out and projecting it onto others. It was like getting teeth pulled one by one over a very long period of time without any anesthetic, but instead of physical pain it was emotional pain. And I never knew when the tooth was going to be pulled or which one.

When I look back on my early years of incarceration, I think medication was an easier way for the institution to deal with people like me rather than taking the time to understand me. Also it was unusual, even unheard of for someone with my diagnosis to work on recovery without medication. When I talked to staff about the simplest things, I found myself expressing the words with great intensity as I struggled to get them out. I wanted so badly to be heard and understood. Not being on meds, the intensity of struggling to get the words out along with my history understandably created anxiety for the staff. My efforts to be understood probably came across like I was angry and about to do something rash. I was just trying desperately to get them to hear me. I felt like the character Festus on the 1960s TV series called *Gunsmoke* that starred James Arness as Matt Dillon. When Festus was trying to get people to understand him, he would keep repeating, "Don't you see? Don't you see?"

Roughing it for me was going to bed many a night in so much emotional pain that water leaked out of my eyes, but I couldn't cry. It meant having dreams where I was on my back paralyzed with suffocating emotional pain that made me feel like I was dying as I struggled desperately to wake up.

I was once told that part of the healing process was that you get worse before you get better. And I indeed experienced that. I had lived with fear for so long that it became my natural emotional state. To feel at peace or safe was frightening for me. It felt dangerous. I knew I must be missing something. I could be in my room with my door closed and hear someone next door talking to someone, and I would be absolutely sure it was about me. I could be walking the hall and others would be walking the hall, too, talking to each other. I would pull anything out of these conversations that came across as threatening or a putdown and take it as though it was directed specifically towards me. How could I get to a healthier and better way of being and of doing life if I could not imagine what this different life would look like? I only knew a daily life filled with being constantly on guard against threats.

Stage 1

After a year and a half, medication-free, I was moved from a maximum to a medium security unit. Some staff on maximum security passed on to the staff in medium that I seemed better on meds. Seems to me that could be said about a lot of people ill or not!

Soon after arriving, the new unit manager came to me and said that he wanted me to share all my thoughts and feelings. I initially resisted. It took me awhile to figure out why. I think I was fighting against two things in my past. First, because of the physical abuse that I suffered as a child and being told to shut up when I cried while being beaten, I got a strong message not to talk and that my feelings do – not – matter – period! The second thing I had to fight against was my earlier training as a young adult man to keep my feelings and thinking hidden. Men were considered manly if they appeared strong and silent. Revealing my thinking seemed dangerous as it gave others an advantage over me. Revealing my feelings made me feel vulnerable and weak. The decision to share my thoughts was a huge step in the recovery process.

I went from hardly ever sharing my thoughts and feelings to letting them all out. That was the first time anyone wanted to hear what I had to say. So much came out of me. I found myself stopping and talking to any staff that would listen. I was elated. Eventually they assigned a staff to me because some of the staff had a hard time handling some of the things I shared.

Getting all that stuff out of me worked like magic when it came to my recovery. I learned and experienced that when I talked to a caring person about my fears, anger, shame, sadness, and pain, the power of these emotions over me started to decrease. For the first time I started working to feel and recognize my emotions and discovering my emotions didn't dictate my actions. My actions were my choice. Wow.

The unit manager who asked me to share all my thoughts and feelings strongly held the opinion that I should be on medication and still thinks so. I believe he wants what he honestly thinks is best for me. In thinking about medication, if I had received a prescription and dosage that worked for me and my illness at the very beginning before I had those bad experiences, I believe that medication could have assisted my recovery in the short term. Still, I prefer the medication-free route I've taken. This institution considers medicating for mental illnesses like mine to be a life-long solution, as many (if not most) institutions believed at the time I entered and still do.

This same unit manager also said that he never met anyone who works as hard as me to understand himself. He will say that even to this day. Yet, he's not able to accept my recovery without medication. The persistence of his opinion and my respect for him led me to never take my healing process for granted. I knew my recovery had to be real and rock solid. By rock solid I mean genuine recovery. I had to be free of delusions and so I have to be aware of and in control of all my feelings and thoughts including any kind of fear, anger, or hatred. It means to understand what is happening within me all the time. Put another way, I had to learn about and understand the things that played a part in my becoming ill.

I remember him once saying that he understood me wanting to get healthy without medication. He went on to say that there were two other patients he knew who also felt that way but that they ended up on meds anyway. All I could think of at the time was, "I am not them." I didn't know those two people, but I do know that people have different levels of resolve about different things. I felt relentless determination to be medication-free and, even more importantly, I discovered a realistic plan. In addition, I developed a deep knowing that without the belief of something greater than my illness, I didn't stand a chance of recovery. Without knowing the two other patients' level of resolve or spirituality, I couldn't compare myself to them and their situations.

Several years went by and I didn't give a lot of thought to being ill. When it came to being what is called normal, I didn't have much of a reference point. Illness was my normal. Then I began having moments of a different feeling; times when I felt good. Without realizing it, the fear was gone. The difference between what I was used to feeling—self-conscious, worthless, and suspicious—and what I was feeling in those moments was like night and day. Picture someone alone and afraid, huddled in the dark protecting his head against the next blow. Now picture someone running along a beach on a sunny day, filled with excitement as the gusting, swirling wind lifts the kite he's flying in all sorts of directions as it flies higher and higher.

In those brief moments of lightheartedness, unrealized at the time, the fear was replaced with fearlessness and openness to life. Early traumatic childhood abuse can rob people of innocent spontaneity. I had learned to live my life always on guard because if I let my guard down and I was harmed it felt so much worse than if I stayed vigilant. Eventually it started to seem as if letting my guard down *caused* something bad to happen to me. I learned to live my life alone, never trusting anyone, always fearful and watchful.

One day I was having one of those surprisingly good feelings. I felt great. Without realizing it, the fear was completely gone. In the entrance of the small dayroom on the floor was a towel that I didn't see. I was wearing shower slippers and when I pulled open a heavy metal door to enter, my foot touched the towel and its softness startled me by the unexpected sensation and the change of sensation from heavy metal to soft material. I quickly became vigilant again and retreated into my paranoia where I would be safe. These initial brief moments of lightheartedness, when I was unaware of my guard being down, were difficult to come to terms with because the shift back to vigilance felt so extreme. It was like being on military guard duty and falling asleep at your post without knowing that the enemy was sneaking up on you. Suddenly you awake with the realization that you are surrounded. You foolishly allowed yourself to be trapped.

The experience with the towel let me know without question that I was very ill. It also taught me on an intuitive level that recovery was going to be a long journey. Before that towel, I thought I was pretty much okay. From my perspective, nothing really stood out to me to make me think I was ill. I made sense of my world and my reactions to it. The mundane experience of the towel was so jarring that I could finally see for myself that I was very sick. I started to understand that I had developed patterns of odd thinking to make sense of experiences that were really part of my illness. I finally just knew there was no way for me to simply think my way through this. There would be no magical healing.

I don't matter; I am worthless; no one loves me; no one respects me; I'm a bad person; I'm no good; I don't count; I don't deserve. What all these expressions and others like them have in common is that any one of them can create unbearable pain and suffering. I was terrified of feeling the pain of worthlessness and more so of others finding out how I felt about myself. My recovery has been about acknowledging and facing head on the fear of these painful emotions.

The idea of *unresolved issues* has helped me to understand how I became so ill. As a child I had no way of understanding how to deal with those hurtful, painful, and fearful injustices I experienced. So I ended up with a choice of either believing them or trying to suppress them, filling me with self-doubt about my worth or burying them to grow and come to the surface at unplanned moments. They became unresolved issues (unfinished business), which meant that although those hurtful issues were in the past, they still affected my life in the present. They affected every area of my life. They affected my relationships, my thinking, feelings, and actions. On subtle and non-subtle levels, my basic emotion became fear, fear, and fear.

Through the years the unresolved emotions continued to manifest in my dreams. In one dream I had here at the institution, I was with some friends I used to sing with in high school. As I was remembering and experiencing the joy of those warm moments of long ago, in an instant my friends disappeared. I was overtaken with deep sadness and started to cry but couldn't. The emotional pain intensified so quickly I couldn't breathe and my heart felt like it was about to explode. I lay paralyzed from the fear, yet struggling desperately to wake up.

Two Gifts

On the PBS TV channel, a series was shown by a gentleman named John Bradshaw called *Reclaiming and Championing Your Inner Wounded Child*. That was gift number one. Some of the men and women in his audience were holding stuffed animals. Bradshaw went on to explain how the stuffed animals helped them to access the feelings of the wounded child within them. I was so taken by the program and so serious about recovery, I decided I wanted to get a stuffed animal, too. I wanted a Teddy bear. I was in my 40s at the time and fortunate to have a therapist who understood the inner child concept. He had recently come to work at the institution temporarily. He was gift number two.

The Bradshaw series along with my therapist helped me to understand my illness for the first time in a more concrete way. Up to that point, unlike a physical illness where you could say my arm hurts, mental illness was very unclear to me.

One day the therapist said to me, "Louie all of you is not sick. You have some good parts and values; you just have to claim those values." He went on to say, "Pretend that this little 5-year-old is standing in front of us and it is you. This little boy is the sick one and doesn't trust anyone not even you. Your job as an adult is to parent him, learn to love him, and bring him back to health, and you can't fool him."

I almost gasped. To hear that mental illness was not all I was was a new idea, one that opened a window to hope. In that moment, my understanding of this mysterious illness of mine became a bit clearer. I was very excited. The inner child work played a huge part in jumpstarting me on the road to recovery. Finally, at last, I had direction, a plan, and it was time to go to work. First thing was to buy a Teddy bear to access the child within and to start resolving those past wounds.

When I told my therapist about buying a stuffed animal, he said it was important to let the staff know. We didn't want them to think I was going off the deep end even more! When the Teddy bear came, I named him Little Louie and a friend of mine even made a yellow shirt for my bear with the name Little Louie on it.

On that first day, I was standing by the closed door in my room holding the Little Louie Teddy bear getting ready to come out and walk the halls. None of my peers were aware of my plan. I was afraid of what others might think. I imagined them saying, "Will you look at that nut case walking around with a Teddy bear in his arms." I was coming out of my room no matter what they might think. My recovery was far too important.

I opened the door. I came out with my head down and one arm around the Teddy bear. As I walked up and down the hall for several minutes, I started perspiring. I only glanced up once or twice. After about twenty minutes of walking, I entered my room and shut the door to contemplate the experience.

The experience brought to the surface the shame and guilt I had been living with for so many years. I saw day one as a success. As time went by, I never really got comfortable carrying around my Teddy bear, but it did become easier. I sometimes stopped and talked to my peers and explained what I was doing and why.

I remember having deep feelings of injustice once when the staff took away a privilege that I had earned. They said at the time it was because they didn't know how I dealt with stress. The privilege was being able to go out of the building to another building for food service. The feeling of being wronged was very intense. Later on about 3:00 the next morning, I awoke still feeling the pain of the injustice. I had a keyboard at the time, so I got up and started puttering around with it as I continued to think about the injustice. I started playing with the inner wounded child concept. I said, "I love you Little Louie." I got very quiet as I thought about what my therapist said about not being able to fool the little guy. As I sat there being very quiet listening for an inner response, I realized that I did not love Little Louie and the tears began to fall. I then said, "But I'm going to learn how to love you." That was the beginning of an honest healing relationship with me.

When I walked up and down the hall with my Teddy bear, I could still feel kind of macho because I only had one arm around him, not two, and because I knew I was in the role of protector. I had little inner dialogues with Little Louie as I walked. I silently said things like, "I love you. You're doing a great job. I'm proud of you. It is safe to express any thought or feeling that you want to me. I won't let you hurt anyone or anyone hurt you." Talk about opening up Pandora's box. All types of violent thoughts came up whenever that child in me felt threatened.

As overwhelming as those thoughts and feelings were at times, I kept assuring that little boy that I would keep him and others safe, too. One day, I don't remember what triggered it, but as I was walking the hall feeling upset, Little Louie pretended to shoot everyone that he saw that he didn't like. I told my therapist about the experience, and he said when that happens that I, as the adult, should take the bullet out of each person shot. I thought that was a great idea.

What I realized was that I had been treating myself (Little Louie) the same way I felt I was treated as a child. I truly had become my own worst enemy. Ignoring and suppressing those unresolved emotions of fear, anger, and hurt kept me emotionally trapped as a child in an adult body.

Something unexpected happened one day as I was walking up and down the hall holding the Teddy bear with one hand and saying positive things to Little Louie. I got an inner response that went like this, "If you love me, put both arms around me." As if I wasn't already embarrassed enough, the thought of putting both arms around a Teddy bear in public out there in the hallway sounded even more embarrassing. Little Louie was more than just a stuffed animal. Little Louie the Teddy bear represented my wounded inner child. Another moment of truth had arrived. Was looking macho more important than showing love for Little Louie? I not only put both arms around Little Louie, I took it a step further. I held the Teddy bear's cheek next to mine. I became a little emotional hugging myself through a Teddy bear. And this was just the beginning. Tough times were still ahead for me.

As the paranoia and stress of constantly interpreting what was going on around me started taking its toll, for the first time I was seriously thinking about taking medication. I was suffering so much. I didn't realize that my first major breakthrough was right around the corner.

I was probably just a day or so away from asking for the medication when a new patient came on the unit and was moved right next to me. Because this person reminded me of one of the men I killed, the stress increased. I thought at the time that this was being done on purpose by the institution to make me suffer and cause me to act out. Then they would have a reason to get that court order to medicate me.

In the beginning, for the most part my new neighbor and I got along. He always told me that if his music ever got too loud to let him know. I didn't realize at the time I was suffering from a degree of Post-Traumatic Stress Disorder (PTSD). I had spent my whole life being on guard from the childhood beatings. If I could hear his music, it was always too loud. I was constantly knocking on his door asking him to turn it down. He started becoming agitated with me, and I with him. I felt our music should not be so loud that the other person could hear it in their room, especially at night when it was time to sleep. He played his radio all night.

Whenever I knocked on his door and he opened it, his music never seemed that loud. I couldn't stand to hear it even a little. There were times when I put my ear up against the wall just to see if I could hear his music. If I heard it, I became irritated. I even reported it to the staff, but they said we needed to work out our differences.

I was trying to reason with myself regarding the situation. I couldn't understand why I couldn't let it go. My neighbor even said we had to learn to put up with each other. On the surface, what he said made perfect sense, but I couldn't let it go no matter how much I tried to reason about his comments and with myself.

It was about 3:00 one morning. I awoke suddenly for no apparent reason and felt instantly awake. I faintly heard his music.

My therapist told me that little kids use terms like, "It isn't fair." Anyway, I had had enough. I got up mad as hell and started pacing in my room. At 3:00 in the morning, I was ready to go over there and smash his radio. I was so full of rage. I remember thinking that if fifty men congregated outside my door with guns and knives, they would be the ones in trouble and not me.

I somehow knew something inside me was in trouble. I didn't have the words for it then, but something was out of whack—out of proportion. I picked up Little Louie as I continued to pace. I kept hearing the words from within, "It isn't fair, it isn't fair." I countered with, "I know it isn't fair but we have to get along." Back and forth the inner dialogue went. All of a sudden in my mind's eye, I saw my dad beating me as a child. I stopped and fell against the door as I continued to hold Little Louie, and the tears started flowing from deep within my gut. I was making a gasping sound as though I had something in my stomach that was being forced out. The whole crying experience lasted only a few minutes give or take, but those few minutes were a profound healing process.

After that experience, his radio never bothered me the same way again. The high and intense fear level I had been living with came down a significant notch. It was enough for me to hold off taking medication. The incident gave me a little more confidence, hope, and even more insight into my illness. This first major breakthrough was just the beginning of many challenging adversities that took place through the years. Although far from being set in stone, my goal to stay medication-free was on its way to becoming a reality.

About a year later, I was confronted with the next major test and opportunity to deal with another unresolved issue related to my dad. There was a big guy on the unit that had a bully-type mentality. I remember feeling intimidated by him. As I thought about what to do, I knew acting out was out of the question, especially if I didn't want to end up on medication. As a small child, my father appeared big to me and in many ways he was like a bully projecting his brutality onto me.

For this big guy on the unit, I came up with plans A, B, and C. In plan A, if he bothered me in any type of way, I planned to pull his chair out from under him while he was sitting on it. In plan B, I would throw a chair up against the wall next to him. Plan C was to ask to be moved off the unit temporarily. I decided to ask to be moved off the unit. The other two plans were not acceptable to me. A staff member who I really liked thought I could handle things without being moved off. Moving off would have meant starting all over earning privileges in the level system once I returned. I didn't want to chance it, so I ask to be moved. Because of what happened after I left the medium security unit to go to a maximum unit, I'm glad I followed through with the transfer. To me, it was important to work through my feelings as far as what that peer was triggering. So I thought out of sight, out of mind.

When I came onto the max unit I was put into a secure room. Evening was approaching so I settled down on a mattress that was on the floor. As I rested feeling my feelings about what had happened on the other unit, I started losing my breath. Breathing became harder and harder by the second. I truly thought I was dying. I didn't panic. I just lay there set on dying.

Then all of a sudden my breath started returning. I got up and started crying profusely. I noticed that I was walking around confused and the steps that I was taking were like that of a small child. I knew I was purging emotional pain from my past. When I returned to the unit a week or so later, I no longer felt threatened by the bully.

The End of the Force

In March of 1995, I had a delusion and I thought the Force wanted me to take the life of one of my peers. I tried to solicit another one of my peers to get a gun. That peer reported me. Because I answered all questions honestly and truthfully, including that no one else was in danger, I was transferred from one medium security unit to another medium security unit. Understandably some staff didn't agree. They felt I should have gone back to a maximum security unit rather than another medium unit. The medium security unit I went to felt like my "home" unit because it was my first medium security unit after I moved from maximum security. My therapist charted the following in my medical file (1995) about the gun incident:

Louie is a very complicated man who presents material openly which most other patients with the same ideation would conceal. If he continues to talk openly with staff I believe dangerousness decreases significantly. Louie's words have always been reliable in the past and he has given his word that no one is in danger.

Because of my commitment to become a healthy person and because of that gun incident, I went deeper into therapy than I had ever gone before. That serious incident became a huge turning point in my recovery and eventually led to a break from my delusional thinking.

As the delusional thinking started losing its hold, the final break came in the year 2001 when my psychiatrist at the time asked me to write a song about the illness (*The Force*). Months earlier, before being asked to write the song, a very important breakthrough in my recovery was when I came to the understanding that the Force did not come from outside me. It was inside of me all along. *I was the Force.* The Force was made up of all those suppressed, painful, frightening emotions I tried to escape from all those years. I had been running terrified from myself.

At that point in my recovery, I had come so far that the writing of the song was completed in a couple of days. It was like it was right there waiting to be written. I did feel some nervousness over letting the Force go. After all, it had been my protector. I felt the Force always kept me from getting caught, and it gave me this strong although uncomfortable sense of purpose, as crazy as it was. This sense of purpose covered up my sense of worthlessness, creating an extremely distorted way of thinking.

Writing that song was the final deathblow to the Force because it violated its most basic and powerful principal—secrecy (its fear of exposure). I not only wrote a song about it, I shared it over and over with others. Every time I share that song, I am choosing health over illness. The only thing the Force could do, was die. The whole existence of the Force and its power depended on that secrecy. I was the only one who could expose it. The Force was like a vampire brought out from a dark cave of delusions into the sunlight. It couldn't exist in the clarity and reality of the light of day.

The components that made up the Force (the delusion) were intense fear, incredible anger, and devastating emotional pain. It was only when I found the courage and strength to start facing these emotions by feeling them when activated by some perceived injustice or something someone said or did or just thoughts popping into my head related to any of those emotions that the Force began to die. I discovered that one key for me was to not project my feelings on to someone else. Only then did I start to find my center and regain control of my actions. Every time I dealt with an emotion by feeling it and not acting on it, the Force little by little, month after month, year after year, disintegrated and the light shone in its place. That light was clarity showing that the real me was more than the horrific things that I had done.

Chapter 6

Recovery after the Force

I had a strong sense as I was coming out of my delusion that now I was going to have to deal with the raw emotions of fear, anger, and hurt that I had suppressed for all these years. I had been fighting a war and the Force had been my protector, my adversary, and my rationale. I would now be fighting a different type of war—a conscious inner war with myself, where it all started in the first place. As much as I knew that vanquishing the Force was the right and healthy thing to do, I also knew that it would leave behind a hole that I wasn't sure I knew how to fill.

Living with Emotions

Early in my recovery process, a therapist said, "Whenever you get angry, Louie, ask yourself, 'What am I afraid of?'" I had never thought about the relationship between fear and anger. Because of my commitment to understand what had happened to me and what I did, the therapist's words demanded exploration. Honestly, I could not think of one time out of the countless times that anger appeared in my life that fear was not present to some degree.

The fear attached to my anger was generated by low self-esteem, lack of confidence, and a sense of general worthlessness. Worthlessness carried a huge weight of shame, pain, and hurt on its back. Once I accepted this new knowledge about myself, I had to struggle to befriend these emotions and see them as allies. I needed to regard them as beacons guiding me through the treacherous, stormy waters of insanity to recovery. Facing these emotions, becoming aware of the thoughts that triggered them—untrue thoughts about who I truly was—and learning to move through them rather than to be paralyzed and controlled by them was one of the greatest challenges I ever faced. Worthlessness – Fear – Anger – Delusions. The reward of maintaining the personal balance I have learned and achieved is that the delusions do not go spinning out from the emotional chaos. And my thoughts then have a chance to organize themselves in a healthy way.

When under the influence of the Force, any hint of hurt, fear, or anger could trigger delusional thinking. Nothing could be taken at face value. Everything had a message of some kind in it. Was it just in my mind or was the Force truly gone? It didn't take long for that test.

After being moved to the other medium security unit, a breakthrough paranoid incident took place. A fairly new patient who I liked as a person came to me one day concerned about being called in to see the staff because of an inappropriate remark he felt he might have made to a female staff member. I gave him the best advice that I could and forgot about it.

The next day something happened that caused me to feel threatened. I started becoming paranoid. Now normally paranoia led to me becoming delusional. The inner work I did regarding the gun incident and the writing of the song about the Force had moved me away from becoming delusional and made me strong enough to face and work through my emotions a little better. Of course there was obviously work still left to be done in that area of my life. When I thought about the Force (my illness), I thought about how I could respond to different situations rather than acting on them.

Anyway, as I sat in the dayroom pretending to be reading the newspaper, I felt the anger and paranoia creeping in. I saw certain peers and felt they were part of a conspiracy to threaten me in some way if I didn't act a certain way. These peers were people I liked and got along with. Once again the Force was letting me know that it would hurt me in some way if I didn't act the way it wanted me to. This time I was fighting back against the Force by allowing myself to feel my fear and anger. I was determined there would be no acting out on any delusional thinking this time.

As I sat there—now pretending to read the newspaper—I was steaming with anger at the thought of others threatening me. The peer who had approached me the day before concerned about the inappropriate remark approached the area where I was sitting. He picked up a part of the newspaper and stood right by me reading it instead of sitting down in the open chair. I immediately felt he was also part of the conspiracy.

My anger got even stronger. I thought, "How dare you threaten me after I tried to help you. I thought you were a friend." I wanted to jump up and tear him apart, but I was determined not to act out. After a while he moved away from me. I eventually got up and went to my room still feeling upset. A couple of days went by, and I no longer felt threatened. I decided to do some reality checking. I asked the peer if he remembered standing by me reading the newspaper a couple of days earlier. To my surprise he did. I asked him, "What was going on? Instead of sitting down at the table you stood right by me?"

To my astonishment, he said he wanted to share with me the results of the incident with the female staff. Because I was reading the paper, he said he didn't want to disturb me. He went on to say nothing became of it. I told him I was glad. Shortly after, I went to my room. As I thought about how I had wanted to tear him apart two days earlier because I just knew he was threatening me at the time, I began to cry. Just think if I had acted on my suspicions thinking I was so right, when in fact I was so very, very wrong.

Another test was on the horizon. I found out one day that there were two peers who were bad mouthing me behind my back. I could hardly contain my anger at the thought of it. One day they were both sitting in the dayroom by themselves. I went into my room and pictured myself going in the dayroom and beating the hell out of both of them. As I sat there intensely struggling with my emotions, I told myself to just feel my feelings of anger. I knew to attack them might feel good in the short run, but it would end up being very bad for me. Somewhere in my mind I believe the risk of ending up on medication helped me keep control of myself long enough for deeper feelings to surface.

While sitting there feeling the anger, it started turning into hurt and then sadness. As tears came, I thanked my Higher Power for the tears. I was releasing the pent up pain and anger. I got through it, and I felt proud. My tears were a sign of strength and not weakness. To hurt them in any way would surely have been a sign of weakness on my part. As different events brought out my hidden anger through the years, there were times I felt so angry that to not hurt someone made me feel crazy.

Looking back into my childhood and remembering the terrible hurt and anger I felt in my family, the beatings by my dad, feeling like I didn't matter to my mom, being demeaned and laughed at by my siblings, it all made sense. I was becoming strong enough to finally feel and work through the unresolved emotions without striking out.

Courage. An important and powerful word. To face and overcome my endless fears was going to take courage. To claim my values, to go deep into myself, and to seek out the things I did not want to see or feel, let alone let anyone else see or know about, was going to take courage. To feel my hurts instead of acting them out was going to take courage. To admit when I was wrong was going to take courage. To say to those I cared for and trusted that I was scared was going to take courage. To learn to trust was going to take courage. To accept that in spite of my transgressions I am a good person who cares about others was going to take courage. And finally, to conduct myself in all areas of my life appropriately to the best of my abilities was going to take courage.

Seven years later, I was on the whole doing well, however, the unit psychiatrist approached me one day and said he wanted me to try a fairly new medication. He went on to say if I didn't like it I could stop at any time and that it had very few side effects. Up until then, I hadn't been on medication for a little over seven years. Although hesitant, I agreed to try it.

I was very sensitive to any kind of stimulant. After two days of feeling very subdued and not liking it, I had had enough. I felt like I wasn't fully present. He tried to persuade me to give it a longer try and said that usually to give it a fair try one should stay on it for at least six to eight weeks, but I was having none of it. I had come too far to sabotage the work I had done and start depending on something external to control me. I was more convinced than ever that the path I was on was the right one for me, and it would be just a matter of time before I would know without any doubts that I would be able to fully function without the aid of medication. So the journey to be medication-free continued.

Women

Each adversity I encountered and handled appropriately brought me closer to wholeness. One of the problems the institution—probably most institutions—ran into from time to time was a peer and a female staff member becoming overly involved with each other. Sometimes such a situation ended up on the local news. As the months and years continued to pass by, I found myself sometimes becoming attracted to a female staff member. I did not want to become the subject of the 6 o'clock news hour. I thought it best to be aboveboard and transparent about my feelings. I thought it important to stay appropriate and to keep things in the light.

I didn't have a good role model growing up. My dad, who was separated from my mom, ended up having three different women in his life. So when I found myself attracted to two female staff members on my unit, I thought about my dad having those different ladies in his life and wondered if I could possibly be acting out what I saw in his life and character. I decided to treat my feelings for these women as an opportunity to learn more about myself and grow from the experience. I respectfully told each female staff member how I felt about them and the other staff member. I also told them how I thought I was mimicking my dad and that this was an opportunity for me to move beyond my early upbringing.

I really did not have the past experiences or social skills to know how to handle situations like this. I thought my plan was a good one, a respectful one, a healthy one. I thought I was doing the appropriate thing. Because of my history, some staff members had an understandable fear of me and I was not always taken the way I intended. The female staff members who understood my dilemma—either be secretive about my feelings which was not encouraged by the mental health team and would prevent my growth in this area or tell my feelings and risk being misunderstood—helped me greatly to heal from the terrible fear I had regarding intimacy.

I asked both ladies if they minded me going to the team to make them aware of what was going on. The team is made up of the staff on the unit and you could ask to meet with them all at the same time. They both said it was okay. I was excited. I went in and told the team how I felt about the two female staff members and that I knew I had to be appropriate in my communication and contacts with them. I told the team about my dad.

One of the nurses complimented me for my honesty. She went on to say other men might have tried to act on their feelings. Her praise made me feel good and reassured me that I was doing the right thing. I started becoming more spontaneous and gaining more confidence in myself. It didn't last long, though. From my point of view, although I remained appropriate, both female staff became uncomfortable and in my opinion started takings things out of context.

For example, there was only one hallway on the unit; everyone passed that way. When one of the female staff members arrived on the unit, I was accustomed to cheerfully greeting her. She told the other staff that she felt like I was waiting for her to come on the unit. Like I was stalking her. It wasn't like that to me, and I didn't know what to make of it.

Eventually I was moved off the unit. My confidence was shattered. I felt so hurt. I thought I was getting a handle on behaving appropriately and doing the right thing. It really brought me up short.

On the new unit I was very quiet. When talking with any of the female staff members, I weighed my words very carefully. You talk about being between a rock and a hard place. That unit's team criticized me for not being spontaneous when talking with the female staff. They said I came across like I was trying to hide something. I had just been removed from a unit for being open and now I'm supposed to behave as though nothing had happened?

Back on the other unit, nursing students from one of the local colleges came during the summer months to spend a couple of months training there. I got to know their instructor pretty well. Several times I had a crush on one of the students, and I always let her know. She would tell me how much she appreciated me letting her know those things. Again it was my way of staying on top of things by keeping it all in the light.

Looking back, I have to say although I was very honest and sincere and meant no one any harm, I can see now where some of the things I expressed could have been seen as crossing the line. Some of it, I finally figured out, came down to whom you were talking to. You could say "I like your hair style" to one staff and she would smile, but if I said the same thing to another staff she would find it inappropriate. It was quite a steep learning curve for me, but I did learn through trial and error. I think now that I may have been figuring things out and learning just like a much younger man has to learn and figure things out. Sitting here in the present moment looking back, isn't it about being mindful and treating all people with dignity and respect?

I have come to believe that it is a normal occurrence for male patients to have feelings for female staff members and as such, the institution has a great opportunity to help us deal with our intimacy issues. I remember one particular time when I think the institution handled just such a situation beautifully. The patient involved was sentenced to the institution because he seriously hurt a woman in a park. He was known for being very violent towards women. Let me be clear that I no way condone what Pete did.

Pete's early home life gave him a bad start in life. I remember him sharing with us that when he was about 4 or 5 years old, his mother took a gun and tried to commit suicide right in front of him and his siblings. The gun didn't go off. Both his parents were alcoholics. Sometimes when drunk, his mom came on to him.

Pete developed deep feelings for one of the nurses who is a very nice lady. When the unit manager became aware of it, he set up meetings with Pete, the nurse, and himself once a week to help the Pete work through his feelings. As far as my knowledge goes, that was rare. I hope it helped Pete and wasn't too uncomfortable for the nurse.

Having a few positive experiences led me to change how I viewed my environment and this change helped me a lot. I started looking at this place not only as a mental institution, but as a university as well. I was in a place where learning was available if I chose to take advantage of the opportunity. This led me to start looking at adversities as opportunities. I have to admit, though, there were times I would say, "Damn these opportunities," but still from a growth standpoint that was the healthiest way to look at and deal with my problems.

Tough Spiritual Lesson

Twenty years ago or more, I started taking some spiritual lessons that came once a month in the mail. The idea was to read them every day or some part of them, and then practice the principles they taught. One such principle said to honor those who irritate you. I never heard anything like that before. The closest thing to that was forgiveness. Although very difficult, practicing that principle became invaluable.

There was a peer on the unit named Sonny who went around telling other peers why other peers were here. It didn't matter if his information was correct or not. It got back to me that he was saying I was here because I killed old and gay people. I was very upset. I thought about the lessons saying honor those who irritate you. Here was my opportunity to practice. I didn't feel like honoring him. I wanted to knock his head off. I practiced anyway.

Once a day we had community meetings. All the patients and staff met in one room to discuss things that involved the unit in some way. I thought this would be a good time to practice one of my new coping skills, which was expressing my feelings in an assertive way. I was feeling uncomfortable but started talking about how I felt it was not right for anyone to be going around telling others why people were here. I thought I did a good job of expressing myself.

There was no mention of who the peer was. Sonny spoke up anyway saying he was the one and that it was his right to say what he wanted because of freedom of speech. Others spoke up against his actions also. It was clear that Sonny did not care about my feelings. After the meeting was over, I walked out so mad that I couldn't talk. As the days went by I kept thinking about honoring those who irritate you. Finally I asked myself a breakthrough question. The question was, "Why did it hurt so bad?" Even though he was incorrect about who I had killed, the fact was I had taken human lives. Sonny's actions brought the pain, shame, and guilt I was living with back to the surface.

Recognizing what Sonny's action was tapping in me helped me make more sense of the idea of honoring those you feel irritated by. I have to admit though, when Sonny left the institution I was a happy man. As I experienced the different adversities that came up through the years, each one made me stronger, just like my experience with Sonny.

Town Trips

In 2002, after fourteen years, I finally moved to minimum security. Over all I did very well. I moved up the level system and got town trips. It had been about seven years since my last town trip. The town trip was to the grocery store and it was especially memorable. There were two staff and three peers.

When I stepped into the store, all of a sudden there were all these people. The unit manager was one of the staff on the town trip. He said something to me and I felt so overwhelmed with the sudden stimulation of it all, I couldn't respond to what he was saying. I was in a panic. I heard his words clearly but I couldn't make out the meaning. It was as if he was speaking in a foreign language. It must have lasted only a few seconds but it seemed longer. I was okay after that. For the most part I really didn't like town trips. Plus at that time, I saw myself as never being free again. Not only did I not want to be free, I thought I didn't deserve to be free.

While on the town trips, we were told to not draw attention to ourselves. That was far easier said than done. We had to stay in a group. We were different races. We dressed differently. Some of us had on institutional clothing. Our affects were different. Some of us looked like we were in a trance. There was one peer who was always talking to himself. I think I was more afraid of being found out than anything else. What would the people think if they really knew who I was? And then there was the staff. Depending on which one was with you, they could be bossy to the point of coming across like they wanted the people around to know they were in charge of you.

Actually the very first town trip I ever took was while I was in medium security. It was under very different circumstances. I had to go to the eye doctor for a check-up. I was put in restraints. On the unit, I sometimes heard some of my peers talking about how bad they wanted to be free again. When I got back from seeing the eye doctor I was very glad. I felt fear all the time I was away.

I continued to be open about my thoughts and feelings with the minimum security staff. Different things came up and I told them what it would have been like if I was still under the influence of the Force. For example, if I was upset over something a peer said or did, I'd share how it would have affected me. What I didn't realize is that certain staff were charting what I said from their perspective rather than how I meant it. Down the road it was used against me.

I had reached the point in the level system where I could now ask for a privilege that allowed you and one or more of your peers to walk the beautiful grounds for up to two hours without a staff escort. This had to be approved by the forensic director. About two months after I applied, I received a note from the director saying although I had little or no problems on the unit, I still could not have the privilege at this time. There had been an escape a few months earlier and this influenced his decision against me. Not against anyone else, just me. Others continued to get that privilege. I was told it would be about six months to a year before I would be considered for that privilege.

When I inquired again after a year, the unit manager told me that because I was not petitioning the courts for release, it didn't make sense to give it to me. My argument, which was to no avail, was that I needed the chance to prove myself like everyone else. What I didn't realize at the time was that the real problem was that I was not on medication. That came out shortly down the road when the psychiatrist at that time said that if I was on medication, people might be more favorable in letting me have that privilege.

One of the challenges that comes with getting healthy is that some caregivers keep seeing you in the past rather than in the present, especially if you're what they call a high profile patient who's not on medication. Part of their understandable way of thinking, especially the administrative staff, is that they will be in big trouble if something happens. It's so much easier for them to keep denying you and not taking that chance no matter how well you're doing.

I've always tried to put myself in the administrative staff's place. I committed the horrible acts that brought me here. I know that I would have the same concerns as the administrative staff if our positions were reversed. Still, if the institution has rules about getting privileges for good behavior, I think the rules should apply to my good behavior, too. I try to look at it clear eyed wondering if I'm thinking about it wrong, but some staff have said encouraging and supportive things to me that make me think that others see that the rules are not the same for everyone, even though I think they are supposed to be. There are times that I feel discouraged about trying to learn and do better and not having it recognized. I feel then as if the kitchen sink was thrown at me, or even as if a lot of kitchen sinks were thrown at me! But then I remember that adversity is my opportunity to learn more about myself.

As the saying goes, "I can't heal what I can't feel or see." To resolve an unresolved emotion meant that I needed to courageously feel that particular emotion to its end without acting out. If I felt hurt by what someone did, said, or some other situation, it meant not acting out with uncontrolled anger physically or verbally towards anyone or anything. That hurtful emotion felt like a fire burning around my chest area. That fire was the pain and fear of that emotion. Staying with that hurtful feeling without acting out or acting out as little as possible gave time for that emotion to burn out and resolve. Sometimes it had to play out over many months in different situations before it became fully resolved. Resolved meant that issue no longer controlled me, and I had developed the coping skills to deal with it.

After seventeen years or so had gone by in the institution, a series of events was about to take place that would either show just how far I had come or not come in my recovery. A peer I will call Roger was very bright and gave me insightful feedback regarding my original music. We had developed a little bit of a bonding while on a medium security unit together. Like me, he was not on medication. The minimum security unit that we moved to had two different living sections that were separated by a door that was locked in the evenings at about 10:00 and opened at 7:00 in the morning. Roger lived in one section and I lived on the other.

Roger could be very nice one second and nasty with you the next. Those sudden changes kept me from wanting to get too close. I could be moody at times, also, but it was very important to me that I treat others respectfully even if I wasn't in a good mood. This was something I had to do a lot of conscious practice with.

When we had our unit picnics, a representative for each side divided up any remaining food for his side. My side had the most people. There was a peer on my side named Ted. Ted was not allowed kitchen privileges because he ate up everything. I volunteered to take him into the kitchen whenever he wanted to eat.

After this one particular picnic, Ted wanted a salad but we ran out of dressing on our side. I went over to the other section to get some dressing. There were two peers in the kitchen at the time. One of them was Roger. I ask the other peer if I could get a little of their dressing. As the peer was approaching the refrigerator to get some dressing, Roger intervened and told the peer not to do it. Feeling a little upset, I explained that I just wanted a little for Ted. He still insisted that I couldn't have any. I told the peer not to pay any attention to Roger and to get some anyway.

Again Roger said no. I then said, "Shut up." Roger said something smart back and I said what are you going to do about it? Roger told me to step into his office, which meant his room. I remember thinking to myself, "Is he talking about trying to hurt me?" I found it hard to believe he would do that over salad dressing.

Not using good judgment, I stepped into his room and with the door half closed he pushed me twice up against the wall and told me to never tell him to shut up again. I just looked at him for a few seconds and said, "You lost it." I then walked out of the room and went to my room. That was the first time anyone had put his or her hands on me since being in the institution.

Those pushes triggered a major unresolved issue of the beatings given to me by my father. As my anger started intensifying, I knew this was going to be a very huge opportunity for growth. The thought of dealing with this in the most appropriate way for healing excited me. The war within me, though, was growing bigger by the moment. What do I do next?

Wanting to not act out was losing the battle as I fought to hang on to the bigger picture. Thoughts raced through my head, emotions continued to intensify, and the feeling that I needed to do something right now became more and more urgent. Fighting hard to not lose control, the last thing I wanted to do happened; tears of hurt began to cloud my eyes. It was a blessing. Out of nowhere came the thought of my victims' families and the pain and suffering my actions caused them. I found myself wishing I could go to the families and apologize for all the suffering I caused them, even though I knew this was not to be.

But then my thoughts went back to the pain and anger I was dealing with in the present. The excitement of handling this in a way that promoted healing and growth was there but the pain and anger of the child within me was steadily growing. I felt this intense urge to do something. Thoughts were racing through my head; I went back over to Roger's section. He was outside his room. I knew in my mind I was not going to hurt him, but I walked up to him and blurted out, "You apologize or I'm going to either have to do something to you or tell the staff." I knew that the "do something to you" part was just a bluff. It was that silly macho trying to act tough stuff.

Roger said he was not going to apologize. I walked away and went back to my room. I decided to tell the staff. Roger denied pushing me. I initially wrote hitting me instead of pushing me. Thinking about that, I realize that even though he just pushed me, to that wounded kid in me the push was the same as being hit by my dad. Although not perfect in dealing with that situation, I survived.

The unit manager put both our levels on hold and began some conflict resolution meetings in which he facilitated. They took place once a week. The first two meetings went well, but I had a hard time with Roger not telling the truth about pushing me. Some of the staff actually thought I was not telling the truth and that I was possibly trying to set Roger up. I made a decision that if at the next meeting Roger's dishonesty continued, I was going to ask that the meetings be discontinued.

At the next meeting, things seemed to be going well. Roger came across pretty relaxed. I felt good myself. Thinking about how much he was affected when I told him to shut up during the incident, I apologized for saying that. I thought about that saying, "It's better to be gentle and kind than to be right." I felt right that day when I told him to shut up but I might as well have been wrong. I wasn't gentle and kind on that day.

We continued to talk. Out of the blue, I asked Roger did he push me when I was in his room. He said, "Yes." My eyes watered as I thought about how difficult that must have been for him to say. I'm sure I felt vindicated, too. Normally peers get sent off the unit for putting their hands on someone. I spoke up and said in the unit manager's presence that it would bother me if Roger was sent off the unit. I know I had no control over that part. Roger did end up remaining on the unit.

Six months after that incident, I was hit by a bombshell when I was transferred back from minimum security to medium. Several things happened right in a row—one, two, three—that caused the setback. I was part of a group that did volunteer work in the community at a place called John's Community Center. We served meals to the needy, and they also had a food pantry. I truly enjoyed the work. We prepared the meals and served them. I enjoyed visiting with the people who came, especially the elderly. I enjoyed hearing their stories about things they did in their lives.

On one occasion a lady I had never seen before was there looking sad and sitting alone. I asked her how she was doing and if I could join her. She was very polite and dignified. We talked about general things and a little about spirituality. It was one of those rare meetings. It was like we knew one another. Then she started talking about the job she used to have as a hospital clerk.

She went on to say how difficult it was to find work and that she was homeless. When she said she was homeless, instantly tears swelled in my eyes and I did everything I could to fight them back but they seeped out anyway. It was in the wintertime and snowing that day. The thought of this lady sleeping in the streets was too much to bear. The reason I related to her in that way was because I remembered sleeping in my car with no one to turn to.

More than likely she was in a shelter, but I thought at the time she was literally living on the streets.

I was determined to help in any way that I could. I didn't have any money on me or she would have gotten it all. I told her the next time I came to the center, I wanted to give her some money. She refused. I explained to her that I was incarcerated, that my needs were being met, and that I felt God wanted me to help in that way. After a while she said she would accept it. I was elated about actually being able to help someone in need. Many times you see advertisements on TV asking for donations, but you wonder how genuine they are.

This felt like the real thing to me, and I was going to play a part in helping someone in need. A month or so earlier I was talking to an elderly gentleman named Roy on a regular basis when he came in to eat. He used a walker to get around. He told stories how he used to fly a duster airplane spraying crops where a mall now sat. He wore expensive hearing aids. I wanted to help. So I asked the unit manager who was at the center with us on that particular day if I could buy Roy some hearing aids. He said I could not. I felt very sad.

This time I was not going to ask. This was an opportunity to help someone I felt was in a crisis. I packed some food in a bag from the food pantry and gave it to her. She left with a smile.

When we got back to the institution, I tried to talk with the staff that regularly took us to the center about the lady I wanted to help. She said she could not talk because of a meeting she had to go to. I wasn't going to tell the staff about the money though. I had a good friend whose wife worked at a hospital so I thought maybe they could find her a job and give her a place to stay temporarily.

The snow was coming down, and I'm thinking the lady has to sleep in the streets. I was desperate to help her. I called my friend and told him about the lady, but he said because other people in need were staying with them at the time they could not take anyone else in. He said he could help with money though. My plan was to talk to some of my peers to see if they wanted to donate some money to help her, too.

Anyway, after talking with my friend's wife later on that day, she gave me a different perspective about helping the lady. She said she would never give money but instead buy them whatever they needed because you never know what they will use the money for. After thinking about that, I remembered seeing her later on sitting with a gentleman that did make me wonder if maybe she was playing me. I mean, she appeared to have someone in her life. I'll never know. My friend's wife probably has the right idea.

The weekend before I was to return to the community center incident number two came up and that incident kept me from returning. A younger peer named Joe came to me one day and said that one of the new peers named Jimmy who had only been on the unit for about two weeks asked him while going over to food service if he ever thought about running off. Food service was in another building, and we usually went outside to get there unless the weather was bad.

Because of Joe's trust for me, his lack of trust for authority figures, and being fairly new to the institution himself, he confided in me. Escapes in the past had caused the institution to shut down temporarily and town trips were canceled. That affected the rest of us. I decided after some thought to let the nurse know what Joe told me, but without giving his name. I said, "A peer reported to me that while going over to food service this afternoon, Jimmy asked him if he ever thought about running off."

Many years ago I was told by the staff that they could not do anything about a peer if information came from another peer because the one peer might be setting up the other. So I didn't do much worrying about it. I didn't know the context of the statement made to the younger peer by Jimmy. I thought it would be checked out and it would be over with.

After reporting this to the nurse on a Saturday, the nurse asked me if I could tell him who the peer was who told me. After some thought, I said I would rather not. The nurse said okay. This particular nurse was also fairly new and very soft-spoken. The nurse conveyed no sense of urgency.

I knew that eventually I might have to reveal that it was Joe but I thought because of his distrust for the staff and his trust in me I had some time to prepare him. When Monday came the other clinical staff would be back, and they would more than likely call me in and at that time I would reveal Joe's name if necessary.

I thought at the time I had done my job by reporting it. The next morning one of the more experienced nurses said that if I didn't tell the name of the peer who told me about the incident and something happened, I could get in trouble. Although a little confusing at the time, it got my attention. So I went and talked with Joe.

I let Joe know that I had to give his name to the staff. He understood my position and was okay with me letting the nurse know who he was. I quickly returned to the nurse to give her Joe's name but to my surprise she didn't want to know. She said I should tell the original nurse when he returned to work for the second shift about seven hours later.

I relaxed again because it didn't seem to be a big deal any longer. My thought was to just wait till the next day, Monday, and wait for the team to call me in. Meanwhile they held Jimmy back from food service. I found that out when Joe approached me and said that Jimmy approached him in anger and accused him of telling on him.

Like me Jimmy was a vocalist and a good one, too. We had talked about music and I shared some of my original music with him. Jimmy was a much younger person, and I thought maybe I could do a little mentoring and put him in contact with some people that might be able to help him musically when he got out. That's why reporting him was difficult. We had started bonding.

Up to the point of telling the nurse about the incident I was proud of how I was handling the situation. I saw myself as being caring and thoughtful but things were starting to get complicated. Now I had the unpleasant task of telling Jimmy that I reported him, not Joe.

I explained to him all the reasons why I felt it necessary to report the incident and the difficulty of doing it. I could tell Jimmy was disappointed. I also said to him that as long as he explained that he was not planning to run off there should be no problem. When Monday came Jimmy was clearly in distress. He came to me several times for advice.

Because a new minimum security unit was being opened at the time, things were more stressful for the staff. Our regular unit manager was going to be taking the job on the new unit. We had an interim unit manager filling in for him. The word downtown, as it was called, where the higher ups hung out was that there was to be zero tolerance.

So Monday was here. The staff was back. Joe and I were outside walking on the patio discussing Jimmy and how we were going to be called in to see the staff. When we went back indoors, to our surprise Jimmy had been transferred back to medium security.

Joe was called in to see the staff team. Then it was my turn. I explained everything in detail and to my surprise I got a level drop. They did not like the way I handled the situation especially when I did not give Joe's name when asked by the nurse. Even after I explained the details, it fell on deaf ears. Joe also got a level drop because he didn't report it. I felt it was harsh. Joe was only in his early twenties and did the best he could. I saw it more as a teaching moment rather than one of punishment for both of us. Had neither one of us said anything, no one would have ever known.

It was now time to go back to the community center but because of my level drop I was unable to go. When they returned back from the community center, the staff responsible for taking us down there approached me and said a lady came up to her and asked for me. When she was told I wasn't there she stormed out of the building. The staff wanted to know what was going on. I told the truth about the money she may have been expecting. I was in more trouble. To be honest with you, I now wish I had said I didn't know what was going on.

Incident three began at the treatment mall, a place we go to where various types of therapeutic groups are held. All the different units meet there just like a college union. You get to see other peers from different units that you might not normally see. When Jimmy was transferred back, I gave him a call to see how he was doing. I felt so bad for him. I recommended that he call patients' rights when he told me they didn't even call him in to get his side of the story. I ended up calling patients' rights for him.

I found it hard to shake off the guilt I was feeling. After a few days I called to let him know I wanted to talk with him at the mall. A buddy of his answered the phone and said he was busy. I gave the buddy the message to pass on to him. A day or so later I went to the mall and Jimmy was sitting down talking with the buddy who had answered the phone when I called. I walked up by them and stood there being ignored. As I waited patiently, his buddy in a passive-aggressive way started using comments like big mouth and big nose. Joe had a big nose and I reported the incident.

When the groups started, they just walked away. I couldn't blame Jimmy for being upset with me. His buddy's comment did not set well with me. It brought another one of those uncomfortable unresolved childhood issues to the surface. The emotional pain I was experiencing was intense, so I knew this was going to mean a big opportunity for growth. I had thoughts of wanting to kill Jimmy's buddy but I also knew that was out of the question. In my almost twenty-three years of being here I had never put my hands on anyone. I was proud of that.

Having those kinds of thoughts though is what made me understand the importance of this opportunity for healing because the thought of wanting to harm someone to that degree was a sure sign of deep unresolved pain and anger. It was going to be hard work. Work that I had gotten familiar with through the years. There was actually a part of me that was excited again because of the healing I knew would happen. Again, the secret was to feel the pain and work through it by feeling it without acting out.

One way I work through this type of pain is by replacing negative thinking with positive affirmations. I also need to realize that the person does not deserve to lose his life. I work to take ownership of my feelings and thoughts without blaming. Sometimes I share what is going on with someone I trust. Staying mindful of this process that could take days or weeks takes commitment. I try to remember that the bottom line is that acting out would be a sure sign of weakness on my part.

A day or two later in the morning, I was in my room reading a book. A staff that I had grown comfortable sharing things with was coming down the hall doing a head count. He opened the door peeked in and closed it. I decided to share with him what had happened and how I was dealing with it. I made him aware of the harmful thoughts I had towards the peer and that there was no way I would act on those thoughts. I also made him aware of the big opportunity this was for healing.

The staff complimented me on how well I was handling things and said that I was doing all the right things. That felt good to hear. A few days later that same staff came back and said that a psychiatrist named Dr. Betters was filling in for our regular doctor. He went on to say he knew Dr. Betters and that he was an okay guy and that I should tell the doctor how I deal with situations. Trusting the staff person, I thought, "Why not?" as this was an opportunity.

The staff came back a few minutes later and said that Dr. Betters was not comfortable meeting with me alone because he didn't know me, but he would see me in a staff meeting. Something didn't make sense to me. Why would a professional psychiatrist be uncomfortable talking with someone who had been on a minimum security unit for over three years and in the institution for over seventeen years? Because I trusted the staff, I overlooked my questions.

Just before the meeting, the staff I trusted said, "Make sure you tell them everything." When I went into the meeting, Dr. Betters, the interim unit manager, and others were there. The staff I confided in sat right next to me.

I went on to explain what happened regarding what I had shared with the staff. After I finished talking, I looked at the staff and said, "Did I say everything?" He said, "Yes." The interim unit manager then said that he appreciated me sharing those things. I had just gotten my level back a day earlier. The unit manager went on to say they were going to hold back my level increase and went on to say because I do such a good job of expressing myself on paper, he wanted me to write down my thoughts and feelings related to the incident and that he would see me Monday.

I didn't understand why my level needed to be held back especially because the peer I was talking about was in a different building, but it was just over the weekend, so I could live with it. I spent the next couple of days writing about the incident and time stamping my thoughts and feelings. It was a very therapeutic thing to do.

I saw the peer I was upset with over at food service during the noon and evening meals. I was still dealing with a lot of anger towards him. His unit sat in seats parallel from us at food service, about 5 feet apart. I usually sat in the same spot every time I went over. He sat down a ways from me. To deal with my pain and anger and the silly thought of wanting him to know I wasn't afraid of him, I purposely sat in a spot that was almost directly across from him. I never looked at him at any time. I did this a couple of different times. Although it was immature of me to do it, it still was helpful in my process. I wouldn't be surprised if the staff noticed my seat change.

When Monday came I had completed the work the unit manager asked me to do and looked forward to meeting with him and getting my level back. When I saw him, he said he had a meeting to attend and that he would meet with me the following day.

The following day I was called in to a team meeting. I gathered the work I did and went in. The interim unit manager and our regular unit manager along with Dr. Turner, our regular psychiatrist, and others were there. Before I could say a word, the regular unit manager said I was being transferred back to medium security. As I tried to express my feelings, I was met with hostilities from the interim manager as well as Dr. Turner. I was abruptly told that security was waiting for me.

I asked to not be put in arm restraints and leg cuffs. Denied. They said that was the way all patients returned back to medium security. Even then, in that moment, I saw this as an opportunity to deal with what were in my opinion injustices.

I was put on a cart and driven through the tunnel system. I felt embarrassed. I had done a musical CD, a song and stories CD related to my illness and recovery, and two different videotapes with doctors. Through the years, the strength section of my treatment plan always stated that I was highly motivated when it came to treatment. My peers also saw me as a model patient. Now the model patient was being returned hogtied to a more secure unit.

Simultaneously I felt hurt regarding the transfer back and excited about dealing with this in a positive way. I actually looked at it as a graduation instead of a setback because I would not have handled it this well in the past. I would have become delusional.

In minimum security you have doors but in medium security you have metal sliding grill gates. When we got to the outside of the grill gate to my new unit, the guard complimented me on how I handled it all. He took off the restraints. I stepped onto the unit feeling the embarrassment and pain of it all, and said to myself, "You made it." For me, the way I handled it was another important sign of my recovery. This was just the beginning of the challenges I faced from that point on. My peers looked at me with surprised looks as though to say, "What happened?!" I went straight to the dayroom and sat down without saying a word to anyone and waited to see what room I was assigned.

As I sat there, the unit manager came up and said to my surprise, "Welcome to the unit, we are glad to have you." Someone of authority at a tough time like this had actually said something very caring to me. I had to fight back the tears. Even in this moment I have to stop typing because of the emotions I'm feeling and that was six years ago.

Setback

Some of the staff on medium security thought I should never have been sent back. I definitely agreed because I saw myself as someone you could work with. Regardless of what we thought, I still had to deal with being sent back.

I was also getting a hard lesson in institutional politics. If someone in the position of power didn't like you for whatever reason, they could take any workable situation and use it against you. I want to think that everyone in a position of authority will always behave professionally. Truth is that they are human beings like everyone and as human beings they have their failings and bad days, and make faulty decisions, too.

Putting myself in some of the staff's place regarding how they saw me, I could understand the difficulty. Here was a guy not on medication, something they had been taught to believe was the only way a person could be helped, and this guy committed several homicides.

After three months, I obtained the highest security level on medium and kept it for three and a half years. Most of those years felt like playing tug-of-war with a tiger: risky to let go but risky to hold on. I do recognize that holding on to the highest security level for three years was significant progress, so what do I mean by the riskiness? It felt emotionally risky to let go and step out onto the unknown path of healing but risky to hold onto what I knew and what felt safe but was not healthy. Risky to trust people because people were often negative triggers, but risky not to trust people because people were also the doors to my recovery.

The whole experience became this grueling opportunity to free myself even more from the lingering fear, emotional pain, anger, and feelings of worthlessness and move farther away from my sense of the unfairness of it all. Over time I began to realize that my sense of worth had depended on external things, like others' opinions of me and what I had or didn't have materially. I needed to learn to depend on myself for my sense of worth.

The key to true freedom would come through understanding and working through my fears. Thanks to that liberating question I had asked myself early-on in my recovery, "What happened?" and remembering I wasn't born psychotic, I found the fortitude to endure and to remain medication-free.

The physical restriction was far greater in medium security than minimum security. I felt it even more having had the experience of being on minimum. I watched my peers come and go from medium security to minimum security and in some cases the same individuals returning from minimum—just as I had—and then after spending some time in medium, going back to minimum. All the while I continued to stay in medium without being allowed to advance. It was difficult not to feel discouraged. I had to keep telling myself that my time would come and to recognize the hurt and discouragement I felt and not try to bury it.

I came to recognize that some just found it too hard to accept my healing, especially without medication. And everyone has experiences and fears of their own that influence their thinking. I needed to understand that. Besides, even if I wasn't physically moving forward, on an emotional level tremendous growth was taking place within me.

Life on Medium and Minimum Security: A Comparison

Life on medium security is very different from life on minimum security. Minimum security has three times the space of medium security, along with two separate attorney rooms with computers in them that we could use and twice as many dayrooms with TVs. Personal room space on minimum security is double that of medium, and we could earn unescorted patio time. We could never have unescorted patio on medium security. Being able to go out on the patio without staff was a huge bonus. Many times when I was on minimum security I was the only one using it. The patio on minimum has several large trees. Both patios are fenced in, but on medium the fence is topped off with razor wire and has no trees. As patients earn higher privilege levels on minimum security, we could walk around the beautiful grounds with one other peer and go down by the lake without a staff member for up to several hours.

There are also huge differences for visitors. Medium security is more like maximum security than minimum security when it comes to visitors. On medium security we all meet in one big room. Two staff members are always present. They sit on a raised stage looking down at us watching for people passing contraband. Imagine auditorium seats all linked together in a straight line. You have to twist your body to look at your neighbor to talk. With three or more visitors it is very uncomfortable and visiting really becomes a challenge. Everyone gets kinks in their necks or backs from twisting. Even the visitors complain about how inhumane it all feels.

Compared to medium security, the visiting on minimum is like heaven. Minimum has several different visiting rooms with no staff observing. After reaching a higher security level, our visitors could visit us in our rooms. On minimum we have up to ten hours of visitation available, seven days a week, with no breaks in the time, while on medium during the week it's only three hours, and on weekends it's three hours in the afternoon and two hours in the evening.

In medium security we can order groceries twice a month to cook in the kitchen, but on minimum we can also have groceries brought in by a visitor. We can cook meals for visitors, and they can bring in a cooked meal. After reaching a certain security level on minimum, we can go while escorted to shop for our own groceries every week. We can attend movies, go and have a nice meal at a restaurant, go to some of the state parks for picnics, and go once a year for a home visit. So for me that meant no more family picnics each summer. And no more family gatherings on Christmas that I so much look forward to.

Unlike medium where we have to be escorted to the gym and exercise room, minimum has a pool table, ping-pong table, two treadmills, and weights all right on the unit. I lost all this when I was returned to medium security.

Making It Work

What I can say with all honesty is that the whole experience on medium helped my recovery big time. It made me stronger in so many ways and assured me without any doubts that I had fully recovered in spite of all that had happened.

I've thought about how I got through the humiliation of being sent back to medium security. My simple answer is that it was by understanding the bigger picture. This includes understanding the institution's perspective and keeping my focus on my goals. My two main goals were to have true inner peace in spite of what was taking place around me and to be medication-free.

The path to both of these goals was the same. It was through my emotions and how I dealt with them no matter how hurtful, frightened, or angry I got when the feeling of worthlessness and sense of unfairness got triggered. Acting out in a negative way was out of the question. I constantly reminded myself over and over again through replacing negative thoughts with positive thoughts and using positive affirmations that I was not worthless. Just like a student might study all day for a crucial exam, I spent my days and time working on myself.

Learning how to cry again released the pressure and brought about additional healing. I also cried out to my Higher

Power within me to help me handle extremely challenging emotional situations and to give me the determination to never give up and the belief that these new ways would help. It was about always being mindful and practicing being the person I wanted to be and watching myself slowly but surely become that person.

Every single time I dealt with a situation in a positive way by being responsible for my thoughts, feelings, and actions, I was rewarded with more confidence, fearlessness, peacefulness, and growing love for others and myself. Those rewards increased my courage, hope, and determination. I was growing and learning an inch at a time.

Before I was able to return to minimum security, I had to make my way through all sorts of roadblocks. I had the full support of the medium security staff. Multiple dates for my return back to minimum came and went. I knew that some staff did not wish me to come back to minimum. I treated this as another one of those opportunities to see how far I had come by maintaining a good attitude with staff and dealing with the delays as best I could in a positive, understanding way. I kept my focus on my goals. Finally it happened.

The staff members on the medium security unit treated me with dignity and respect, and recognized how hard I worked. They helped me to feel a part of the human race. Their support was pivotal to me making it through those difficult times.

A clinical staff recently told me that the staff members were divided in their thinking about me. One group thought I was dangerous and that I had never been mentally ill, so that was why I didn't need medication. Another group thought I had worked very hard and the illness was in remission. Many just didn't know what to think.

Out of all the things that helped me recover, if I had to name the one that made it all work and come together, it has to be spirituality. I believe that at our very essence, in spite of all our flaws, there is nothing but pure love. With love as our core, there is nothing we cannot overcome or learn to live with.

After 20 Years, More Tests

They say there are two things you can count on in life—taxes and death. I would like to add, there's always going to be some kind of test. One of my peers, who I will call Walter, presented me with one of these opportunities-for-growth tests. I didn't really care for Walter, and Walter didn't really care for me. When you don't like someone, it doesn't take much to find something to get upset about. On a day when I felt moody, I was standing at the nurses' station getting my two sets of eye drops with a five minute wait in between. After the first set and since no one else was in line, I started having a conversation with the nurse. My folder was lying on the nurses' station counter when Walter came up to get his medication.

Juggling the next set of eye drops and a tissue, I pushed my folder to the far side of the counter to give Walter some room. I then stepped to the side. Walter grabbed my folder and without looking at me said, "Is this yours?" as he handed it to me in one sweep. Anger instantly surged up in me. I didn't like his ways; I didn't like how he handed it to me; I didn't like his tone. I kept my anger in check, but it was there.

I finished up with my medication and walked down the hall to join another peer. We stood by the phone and discussed possibly ordering some food. We were about 5 feet from Walter's room and he came and stood in his open doorway. Something didn't feel right to me. All of a sudden Walter let out a loud burp. It's odd to call a simple burp a confrontation but that was what it felt like. Walter was looking for trouble.

My suspicion was confirmed when I suggested to the peer that we walk down near my room. As we moved away I heard Walter mimic my voice and repeat what I'd just said. I turned and asked if he was expecting a phone call. Walter said yes, and then we engaged in a staring contest. I wanted to deal with the hurt that came from feeling disrespected by hurting him back in some way. I finally just walked away. A war was going on in me between my hurt feelings and my anger.

A few hours later, I saw Walter enter the patient kitchen. I went in and said, "I have always treated you with dignity and respect," but before I could say anything more he interrupted and said, "Just leave me alone." I immediately left the kitchen. The encounter only fanned my hurt and anger.

Handling these feelings all came down to staying with the hurt feeling until they passed without acting out. My courage to face the hurt and strength to not act out was being tested. If I could stay with the hurt, my reward would be healing and more peace in my life. If I didn't and acted out in a negative way, the pain would just be recycled until another event, not necessarily with him, triggered it again. I was determined not to lose this inner battle. This was a big opportunity to practice my techniques and achieve more healing. Rather than continuing to suffer at the hands of these types of events, I was going to have to suffer through this one. It was easier said than done, but doable.

I started using positive affirmations and positive thinking to replace the negative thoughts. I kept reminding myself of my ultimate goal to have joy and peace in my life and that this was my stuff, my hurt, and my pain. As a positive affirmation I might say something like, "I am a good person," and repeat it over and over. Every time I saw him I wanted to hurt him back in some way. Back and forth this went for several days and nights. I expressed some of my feelings to a positive peer. This helped some. He reminded me that, like me, this person was also in pain. I went to sleep and woke up with all this stuff on my mind. I kept going back and forth between thinking positive affirmations and wanting to hurt him back. It was tiring, but I stayed the course and was bulldog determined to win this inner battle.

Finally the break came. My anger, which shielded me from my fear, subsided, allowing the fear to surface. The fear was replaced with hurt and sadness. I just lay in bed and breathed into the pain of my hurt that I was experiencing around my chest area. When I saw him the next morning, the intensity of my anger had diminished greatly. I no longer wanted to hurt him back. I was proud of myself.

I have been dealing with this type of adversity for many years. It hasn't necessarily gotten any easier when it comes up, just familiar. I once read that, "repetition makes the master." When you're incarcerated in any type of institution, the opportunity to practice healthier responses is abundantly available.

A few days later, Walter apologized to me, and I to him. We shook hands. My apology was about coming up and staring at him. Although Walter is a good guy who I wish the very best, he has a tendency to go out of his way to give others a hard time when he's in a bad mood, so I choose to stay away from him. It's great to be friendly towards others, but at the same time, a mental institution is not the ideal place to look for a friend.

The above example would normally be a small matter for a healthy person. As I continue to struggle and make progress, I look forward to the day when such incidents will also be small matters for me. In my recovery process, I have left no stone unturned no matter how small. I've chosen to put myself under a microscope as I have been rebuilding myself almost from scratch. Recognizing and dealing with what may seem like an insignificant matter is not so insignificant for someone who has been ill for so long and who never really learned good coping skills. As an adult, it has been necessary for me to be very patient and take baby steps in my recovery work.

Fear was the number one enemy of my recovery. It also paralyzed my everyday life when I was growing up. I was afraid to take chances because I might fail or to pursue a relationship because I wasn't good enough or to love myself because I was taught that would mean I thought I was high and mighty.

Current Reflection

It was early on Monday, December 24, 2012. As I sat on the edge of my bed, I felt warm and for the most part safe. It was Christmas Eve. On a very deep level, the little kid in me was hurting and conflicted. I longed for a childhood I never had with my family, as I usually did at this time of the year. I also longed for what I did have. It wasn't Mayberry, but it was better than nothing, I thought.

The tragedy in Newtown took place just ten days earlier, and it had been on my mind quite a lot. Newtown is in Connecticut and one of the town residents described it as being like Mayberry. The children and school staff at the Sandy Hook Elementary School in Newtown were all going about their day as usual on Friday morning, December 14th. The children loved life, school, and their teachers. Out of nowhere a very disturbed young man who once attended the same school as a child shot his way through the school's locked doors slaughtering twenty kindergarten children and six teachers. The children were all 6 and 7 years old. He shot his mom before going to the school. Most of the children were shot multiple times. The shooter then killed himself at the school as the police closed in on him.

Like most of us, I was deeply distressed as I followed the story and watched the memorials on TV. I felt like we got to know some of the victims personally as the parents and friends described what they were like. It was so heartbreaking to think of the horror and confusion they must have felt in those moments of terror. Although the adult part of me understands that there was nothing I could do, the little kid in me wished so badly that he could have been there to save them. Being Christmas Eve intensified my sadness and pain.

It's difficult to grasp that twenty-seven innocent people, twenty of them children, were just going about their days when they were gunned down in their school of all places. Like a church or other sacred place, a school is a place where you should feel safe, loved, and cared for. An even more sacred safe place should be a person's home. His mom was in bed and possibly asleep when killed.

What must it be like for the victims' loved ones? What must it be like for *my* victims' loved ones? They have to wake up each day, especially around the most fun holiday of the year, without the ones who they love. I was also reminded of the confusion and terror I felt when I was 6 and 7 years old. I came through it alive, but back then I was always afraid and I felt like I was always dying.

Update: Request for Release

I did not think that I was being treated fairly at the institution where I'd been for over twenty-five years so I decided to petition for release. The institution has certain rules and levels to progress through according to the patient's success. I had had no delusion for over eighteen years and no physical incidents like fighting, hitting, or putting my hands on anyone through all those years. Still, when I followed the institution's rules, I did not receive advancement to the next level. I know many people do not trust in recovery from my type of mental health disorder unless medication is involved. Since I am medication-free, I think some at the institution cannot trust that I have progressed as well as I have toward mental health. I believed there was only a slight possibility that I would be released, but more than that, I hoped the institution would begin treating me according to the same rules as everyone else.

A court date was set for July 11 and 12. This time it would be a jury trial. My attorney thought I stood a better chance than going in front of a judge. I had several months to prepare.

The family members of one of the victims attended just as at previous hearings. Six jurors were chosen from a pool of about forty people. It was the prosecution's responsibility to prove that I was still dangerous. The district attorney's first witness was his court-appointed independent evaluator. Then the district attorney called several law enforcement officers to the stand to review in detail each of my crimes. A sick, paralyzing, hopeless feeling enveloped me. The district attorney brought out pictures of the crime scenes to be shown to the jurors and courtroom on a big screen. I felt so badly for the victim's family. My attorney objected and the pictures were put in the hands of the jurors. Then somehow they were passed to me. Feeling overwhelmed and trapped, I didn't know what to do. I was not the least bit prepared for the crime scenes to be shown or testimony that included graphic descriptions of my crimes. Later, with no objection from my attorney, the district attorney was allowed to put the crime scene pictures on the big screen during his closing arguments. I was devastated. I didn't know where to look.

The change on the jurors' faces was as clear as if they had spoken aloud. How could the jurors not be moved by those pictures? A friend who was at the hearing later told me that when those pictures of the crime scene were put on the big screen for all to see, the victim's sister put her head in her dad's arms and remained in that position. Hearing that, I wished I had not petitioned the court and knew that I would have to make different decisions about going to court in the future. She and her family were traumatized all over again because of my driving desire. All the way around it was beginning to feel like for some this was a sport and winning or losing was more important than getting to the truth of my dangerousness in the present.

It didn't take long for the jury to come back with a not to be released verdict. There was a little celebration between the district attorney and the family members when the verdict was read. For part of me, it was like watching a movie on TV. Only I was playing the part of the villain and not the good guy.

The next morning in the cell, pain started its slow eruption. I now realize that as I achieved mental health, my ability to feel my feelings grew and grew. At my first trial, I did not fully participate. I *could* not fully participate. I was not capable of experiencing feelings. One of the most difficult parts—maybe *the* most difficult part—about recovering from a severe mental illness is coming to realize the pain and suffering my actions caused others and how they have to deal with the brutal loss of their loved ones for the rest of their lives. There in my cell I was engulfed with harsh, painful feelings. I was pain-filled. I started asking and then pleading with my Higher Power to let me die. I had had enough. It was too painful. I knew that God knew my heart, knew how ill I was at the time, but I was worn out and just didn't want to be here anymore. Every cell in my body ached with pain. Tears poured down my face as I sobbed, bent over the toilet hardly able to stand with my mouth open silently screaming and gasping for breath as though something was being dislodged. I don't recall ever feeling that much pain.

I got a very clear picture of why people commit suicide. The emotional pain along with the feeling that no one cares and nowhere is there any comfort for me left me feeling that I am absolutely alone forever. In those moments, I knew there were those who loved and cared about me. And I had a strong sense of purpose that was also guiding me through it all. But just barely. I knew that only recovery from my illness allowed me to feel that degree of pain. I wonder now if some of the pain I was feeling and releasing was related to all my childhood pain, fear, and anger I had learned to suppress from the sense that it was so big that to feel it would mean to die from it.

My attorney did some good things when he spoke at the trial, but in some ways it was hard to not feel abandoned by him. When I got back to the institution, I sent a letter to the judge explaining my intention to petition in four months with the understanding that I just wanted to have a say and offer the victim's family an opportunity to ask me any questions. I felt I owed that family that opportunity since they hadn't had the chance in court.

Ten days have now gone by since the trial. If someone stays mentally ill, I think maybe it can act as a protection against having to deal with or live with the burden of having hurt someone. Of having killed someone. I wonder. I wonder if somewhere some part of me that was hidden way down deep knew that becoming more and more mentally healthy would open me up to the same deep, devastating, suffocating pain that my actions had caused others. That the pain I caused also awaited me? And is experiencing, accepting, and learning to live with this pain the final step of recovery? I get a strong sort of peaceful sense that it might be. If earlier in my recovery I had experienced total awareness of the pain I caused and that awaited me and if I had seen a clear choice, would I have chosen to remain mentally ill?

Looking back at how helpless I felt as the prosecution presented its case. I can't help but think about my victims and how they must have felt. They trusted me, they felt safe, and I betrayed that trust just like I have felt betrayed so many times. There are no adequate words to express the pain and sorrow I will live with for the remainder of my days over what I've done, and the pain and sorrow my actions have caused others for the remainder of their days.

Three different petitions for release have been filed within the last nine years. None of them really had anything to do with being released back into the public. The first petition which was withdrawn had to do with wanting to apologize to victim's family members and the community. The last two were more about wanting to have the freedom to create and record music and to be treated fairly and like the other patients at the institution. I don't know if I will petition again after I have my say before the judge in four months. I am meeting with a therapist to help with processing the experience.

A month after the trial, for the first time, I found myself thinking about the law enforcement officers who were describing in detail what it was like at the crime scenes. We like to think of them as iron men and women when the fact is they are human beings with feelings and they are doing an incredibly difficult job.

I never once thought about apologizing to them or anyone else who was there for what they had to deal with at those crime scenes until now. It had to be horrifying for them and for that I am deeply sorry for what they all had to endure and live with for the rest of their lives because of what I did.

Chapter 7

Integration

What am I like when I am well? I can be bubbly, talkative, funny, and energetic, and I can be quiet and contemplative. My imagination allows me to be very creative in a constructive way. I enjoy solitude because that's when I'm the most creative, especially when it comes to music, which is my passion. I am sensitive and thoughtful of others' feelings. Sometimes I enjoy watching people when I'm out and about in the common areas. I'm very protective of others in a thoughtful way. I try to see the whole picture rather than to overreact to a situation. I enjoy being of help to others. These days I enjoy my solitude even more.

I believe the most powerful spiritual experience that I encountered that helped me to work through my illness, took place at Neighborhood House. The experience was so potent, it infused me and left in me that indelible impression of being loved and cared for. It was as though a dormant seed full of light within me was subtly broken open and with a very quiet inaudible whisper sprouted out the words, "Louie, hey Louie, you are lovable and worthwhile."

Although it took a very long time before I started to believe it, this very subtle awakening was the true beginning of the painstaking, grueling process of countering the negativity, lack of confidence, anger, and self-hatred I was so burdened with. The love and care The Neighborhood House staff gave me in those early formative years was life-saving. They gave me the fortitude to never give up on becoming the best person that I could be no matter how confusing and difficult life became.

A second touchstone from my early years was my mom and dad's work ethic. Their discipline had a powerful if subtle effect on me, too. They always went to work no matter how hard things got.

What the Word Cured Means to Me

Someone once asked me what cured means in my situation. I was a little taken aback and had to think that through because I was making assumptions that cured is cured and means the same for everyone. But it doesn't.

Cured can mean different things to different people. I think of myself as cured but other people don't. They say if I am cured than I wasn't sick before, because there is no cure for my mental illness. They say maybe I'm faking the cure or maybe I was faking the illness. I think of myself as cured, but others think I'm in what they call a remission, like for people with cancer. I do know that my cure didn't happen suddenly, like a virus suddenly vanishing from my body. I do know I have to continuously practice the ways I've found to stay emotionally and mentally and spiritually centered and healthy.

For me, cured means feeling genuine, heartfelt remorse and grief for the horrifying suffering my actions caused so many people. Cured means I am no longer controlled by the paralyzing, paranoid, fear-driven insanity I called the Force. Cured means as a human being I can still experience fear, anger, pain, and even a little paranoia at times. The difference between now and when I was ruled by the Force is that those emotions are no longer my masters. Cured means I can have a violent thought and not feel compelled to act on it. Cured means I am guided by the loving spirit that resides in us all.

I think an obvious question to ask is: What if I chose to no longer believe in that loving spirit? Would I go back into the illness? After all my many fearful years and all the suffering that I've experienced and, even more so, all the pain that others have to live with for the rest of their lives that I caused, why would I ever choose to stop believing in the loving spirit? The loving spirit took me away from that daily hell I used to live in.

The Force separated people into good people who could stay and bad people who had to go. Cured means that I understand that as a human being there's good and bad in us all. Cured means I've become strong enough to claim my life values. Cured means I can hate what someone has done (their actions) but I never have to hate the person. Cured means living a conscious life not an unconscious life. It means living a thoughtful life, a mindful life, a caring life. Cured means caring for all people regardless of who they are or what they have done. Hating an action and hating a person is as different as night and day and makes the difference between living a life of peace and harmony or living a life of turmoil and suffering.

Cured means realizing that I am endowed with free will. I can choose. And to the best of my ability, I will choose love.

Why Am I Confident About My Recovery?

Once I accepted that I was severely ill—which took several years—I wanted to understand how I became so ill and did the things that I did. I didn't and still don't believe I was born with this mental illness. Wanting to know, wanting to heal and become whole again was what gave me a place to start on this journey.

I have had myself under a microscope studying my thoughts, feelings, and behaviors like a scientist for over twenty years. It has become my second nature. I have learned and continue to learn that real power is about taking full responsibility for my thoughts, feelings, and actions, and not power over others.

My recovery has been about being brutally honest with myself. Looking at things I didn't want to see about myself and maybe more importantly, feeling things I certainly didn't want to feel. Unknown to me at the time, I had been running from this all my life. Part of the healing process has been about finding the strength and courage to stop running and learning to feel and work through my unresolved emotional hurts and fears without projecting them onto others. Put another way, it was about learning to take full responsibility for my thoughts, feelings, and actions, and not blaming others for them.

As I mentioned earlier, one caregiver strongly advocated medication for me. I think his position on medication is understandable considering my history, which I can't change. He has said on several occasions that he never met anyone who worked as hard as I do to understand myself and my condition. I spent many days and nights working through agonizing, torturous, emotional pain, and paralyzing fear. From my perspective and experience, you can't do this kind of work for this many years without making progress toward mental health.

In the past it was far easier to become delusional and project onto others than to face my pain and fears. Facing the magnitude of the untold pain and suffering I have caused others and dealing with the personal grief that I continue to experience over what I've done motivates me to become the very best person that I can be. I am no use to others or myself if I continually berate myself for things I cannot change.

Learning to trust others so they can help me has been of extreme importance. Their belief in me has been crucial. For their help I am very grateful because without it I don't believe recovery would have been possible. Most importantly, I believe in and have a Loving Higher Power on board that I look to for gentle guidance.

Presently, I continue to work on things like patience, tolerance, understanding, gentleness, gratitude, self-esteem, and forgiveness of others and myself.

All the above is why I am confident about my recovery. As confident as I am about my recovery, I still have a relapse prevention plan. It is a very important piece. This plan puts my healthcare providers and me in a position to work together, giving added assurance to my recovery.

Full Circle

After three and a half years of being on the medium security unit and holding the highest level for over three years without losing it, I was way overdue for a transfer back to the minimum security unit. Some medium security staff were frustrated and working very hard to make that happen. Some staff on the minimum security unit put up strong resistance to having me back. Many meetings took place between the forensic director and staff of both units. The forensic director said he was surprised at the resistance. There was frustration all the way around.

Most of that resistance from some minimum staff came from the fact that I was not on medication. There are those who believe you cannot recover from a mental illness at all and believe that for sure you have to be on medication for the rest of your life. The institution was and is pro-medication. While I understand the thinking, I just don't agree with it. To me I am living proof that other recovery techniques work, too, when used consistently and with commitment. Sometimes it seems odd to me that some caregiver staff and medical personnel appear to disbelieve in the very techniques and tools they are teaching us.

Through the months I was sent through a maze. The time table for my return kept changing. After months of delays, the minimum unit wanted me to write a letter explaining what the unit could do for me. Everyone knew it was a normal progression to move up through the level system to the least secure unit to show you were making progress. I wrote the letter. When they read it, I was told it wasn't good enough. So with the help of the medium security staff, I wrote another one and got the same answer.

At one point the forensic director said I wasn't as bad as some staff on minimum were making me out to be and probably not as good as some staff on medium were making me out to be. After many disappointments, returning to minimum security was approved. I had to sign an agreement that there would be no town trips for a year and that I could no longer have a patient run business. Losing my music was a huge loss for me.

After a year back and no problems, I put in a request for town trips. To my surprise, my request was denied. Again the main reason was not being on medication. It didn't matter that I never had any physical altercations with anyone or that I was seen as someone who took recovery very seriously or that there were no major incidents on the normal everyday town trips I took before for three years.

As discussed earlier, the process of healing has been about dealing with unresolved emotions (pain, fear, and anger) of the past instead of continuing to suppress (ignore) them. Healing could only take place through resolving these emotions by facing them whenever they were triggered by what someone said or did or some other situation without physically or verbally projecting them onto others in a harmful way. It was either face the pain or continue to relive it over and over for the rest of my life.

Like an onion, I peeled back layers of accumulated emotional pain, dealing with and learning about both the earlier pain and the current situation that triggered the pain. I had a strong sense that eventually a time would come when the final layer would be reached. One does not know how or when that final test or opportunity will present itself. When that time does come, I believe the final layer must be experienced in all its fullness without suppressing, avoiding, or denying the pain, and without acting out. I believe that only then will healing be complete. Once that final layer has been dealt with, more than likely residue or memories of those emotions will still be present. But the power of those toxic emotions will be greatly diminished. They will no longer have control over me.

The Gifts

Another year and a half went by and I decided to try again for town trips. So, I put in another request. At this particular time, I really didn't have a strong interest in town trips. In all honesty, I enjoyed only a couple of the trips during the earlier three years; for the most part they made me feel like I had handcuffs on. We were expected to act and be seen as normal. People couldn't know we were from the institution because of fear of a public backlash. Some very nasty things had been blogged about us on the internet. Some staff also shared with us how some of their friends and family couldn't understand how they could work with people like us.

Whenever someone escaped from the institution all hell broke loose. Media attention exploded, and the institution went into shutdown. Shutdown included no walks on the grounds or fishing. In some cases you couldn't go to your therapeutic groups if they were held off the unit. If a person had a job in the community he couldn't go to that either. As far as having community access again, shutdowns sometimes lasted for over a year. In one case it was two years.

Because of the institution's understandable concerns regarding me, I had worked out what I felt was a win–win situation. The institution had concerns with me not being on medication and the greater price they thought they would have to pay if something went wrong. At this juncture, more important to me than town trips and going out to buy something was the need to show that I could handle town trips as a way to demonstrate that I was ready for a move to a less secure unit in the institution with more freedoms. Just like the difference between medium and minimum security is night and day, the difference between minimum and a less secure unit is even greater.

From minimum, when attending food service, which is located in another building, we first line up, answer to our name being called off, and walk over in twos with one or more staff escorts depending on how many are attending food service. Any number over nine people require two escorts. Sometimes we have as many as twenty-five patients. We have 20 minutes to eat starting from when the last person sits down. After the meal we line up again. The staff does another headcount to make sure everyone is still accounted for and then escorts us back. When we go to our treatment groups also located in another building, the same process takes place.

The lesser security unit allows us to walk over to food service by ourselves. Until we reach the level to walk over by ourselves, we walk over with just one other peer and no staff escort. We can eventually walk around on the beautiful grounds alone. We can have our own key to get in the building and our own phone in our rooms. They even provide bicycles to ride. On the lesser minimum security units, we can walk the grounds with visitors and have cookouts with them. Home visits are allowed. We can make three to four times more money. It was the closest thing to being in the real world.

My request stated that I wanted to have the option of going out only once a month. I would be more than satisfied with that. A small group made up of mostly clinical staff met with me to discuss my request for the trips. I was on a security level that allowed town trips at the time. But that level had been modified to not include those trips for me. The modified level allowed me more freedoms within the building. I appreciated those freedoms. I was allowed to walk over to the other wing without permission or a staff escort. I could use the exercise room on that other wing. It gave me two more day rooms with televisions in them to choose from.

On the minimum security level without the modifications made for me, attendance was required on no less than one trip a week. They wanted me to do the same thing. I explained that a trip a week was more than I cared to go on, and how I wanted to live my life with more purpose. I didn't want to be going out just to be going out. Besides, I thought they would be more comfortable with fewer town trips anyway because of their concerns about me not being on medication. I went on to explain that if I was to ever be released back into the community, I wanted to live my life the same way, going out when there was a need to do so. I was hopeful that with my explanation my request for the option of the one trip a month would make more sense to the staff. I also explained how going on one trip a month would be more exciting and give me more to look forward to. I said to go out once a week for me would be like eating ice cream every day. It would be far more enjoyable eating it once in a while. I like coffee but not every day. I look forward to having coffee once a week or less.

One of the newer staff at the meeting who on occasions takes patients to the YMCA went on to say how exciting it would be to go to the Y from time to time. I explained how I went there the last time I had town trips and it just didn't interest me. Another meeting was to take place in two weeks to further discuss the situation. Meanwhile, I shared my feeling and position regarding what took place at the meeting with one of the aides.

The aide found it hard to believe that I only wanted the option of one trip a month. With vigor, he said, "Look! You're finally going to be treated like everyone else." He wouldn't accept how I felt no matter how hard I tried to get my point across. He even became a little stern about the whole matter. He kept bringing up how I had been treated special long enough. And that people were going to wonder if something was wrong with me if I didn't accept the usual routine for town trips.

The word special came across to me as an odd word to describe how I had been treated through the years. As I tried to understand his usage of the word, I wondered if he might be being sarcastic. I've always thought of special in a more positive way.

I spent the next few days and nights thinking about what all had been said, especially how I now was going to be treated like everyone else. The more I thought about it, the better it felt. I kept thinking, "I'm going to be treated like everyone else. *I am going to be treated like everyone else*," is it possible that finally I'm going to be treated like everyone else? Even though I still preferred the once-a-month idea, the thought of being treated like everyone else felt so good.

While thinking about town trips, something else had popped up. I started thinking about how I didn't deserve to be out in the public. I remember once watching a program where a prisoner who had committed a heinous crime felt he forfeited his right to be back in society. I now understood his feelings even more. Even though I was still ready to attend town trips, I felt even stronger about the option of once a month.

After two weeks, the staff and I met again. Instead of what I thought would be more discussion, they got right to the point and said that I was to attend town trips once a week like everyone else. I went on to say how part of me felt undeserving of town trips and that once a month was just fine. One of the staff at the meeting surprised me when he said, "Because of all the new feelings, your town trip experience may be different than before." This particular staff was someone who had wanted me on medication from the beginning of my incarceration. His words made me feel good and made some sense to me, too. Even though I still didn't feel one a week was necessary, I started thinking about the therapeutic value of going out once a week. I could use the trips to test out the new feelings. I said I would go.

On the less secure unit you don't have to attend town trips. So my thought was that after I got to that unit I could go on trips when I wanted to. The staff did say one other thing in the meeting that made sense to me and that was how they needed to be able to evaluate me to see how I handled the trips. In a week or two I would be on my way. Meanwhile, I was asked to write out what is called a treatment objective plan related to the trips.

The first part of this plan is called Personal Check-in. I needed to make a list of issues I would be working on and share it with the escorting staff prior to going on a trip. For example, "When I'm out on a trip, I will be mindful of my thoughts and feelings." After completing the plan, I was asked to share it with the staff responsible for getting us ready for town trips. When I presented my plan to her, she suggested that I also add in the Personal Check-in section, "It is alright to be part of the group when out." In the past, on my previous town trips, one of the issues brought to my attention was how I needed to stay physically closer to the group.

When she made that statement, "It was alright to be part of the group," immediately upon hearing those words, and I mean all within a split second, I felt panic. A slew of emotions ran through me. I went from initially feeling stunned (confused), to feeling overwhelmed with a spark of joy, then suddenly it turned into sadness as the tears quickly welled up in my eyes, but in a flash the sadness turn to terror. All this happened before you could say, "It's a nice day."

Those words, "It's alright to be part of the group," was like hearing, "Welcome home," or "You belong." As I felt the pain around my broken heart, that statement transported me back in time to those moments when I felt anything but accepted by those

I so deeply loved (my family). I never felt welcomed then. Welcome home was just too painful to hear and accept in that moment. This was my first time understanding why I kept a distance from the group when out on those earlier town trips. I didn't feel accepted. I didn't feel good enough.

When out on those trips, I always told myself that I didn't want to be too close to the group because I felt we looked odd and stood out too much. On an even more honest level that I am a little embarrassed to write, I tried to make it seem like they weren't good enough for me so that I could avoid feeling those unresolved feelings of pain, fear, and anger related to rejection. Without giving anyone a chance, I rejected them before they could reject me. But the truth was I was still living out the feeling of rejection and still trapped in a maze by those painful emotions I felt as a child over fifty years later. And people find it hard to believe that something that happened to them as a child can affect how they see and experience the world as an adult.

Several more weeks went by as I mentally prepared myself for the outings. I started wondering what was taking so long. Once the unit staff approved the town trips, the request went to the forensic director for final approval. We had a new director and I wasn't expecting any problem. I don't think anyone else was either. The staff that worked directly with me and those who knew me best had approved it. When I ask the unit manager what was taking so long he said the trips were now being discussed and in the hands of the institution's administrators. I thought things were still okay and that maybe they were discussing the once-a-month option that I wanted. I thought how great that would be! A couple more weeks went by. Again I asked what was going on. I was told I would have news the following week.

The next week I was playing a card game with some of my peers. The unit manager interrupted the game and said he wanted to talk with me. He said after some more thought and input from other administrators, I was still seen as a risk to the public, therefore town trips have been denied.

Stunned and numb, I went back and finished the card game. Later on, a part of me (the little kid) went from feeling like I was picked up over someone's head with joy, celebrating being treated like everyone else, then suddenly, slammed down to a ground made of concrete with hot fiery nails sticking out. It hurt so bad. Even after all the hard work I had done through the years, I was still not accepted. I was still a bad person. I was still flawed and not good enough.

Looking back at that split second slew of emotions moment, when the comment, "It's alright to be a part of the group" was made, it's fascinating how quickly my emotions mirrored my rapid fire thoughts. It reminded me of two similar incidents. The first incident took place over forty years ago. I was in my early twenties at the time. I was going out on a date with a very nice lady. An associate introduced me to acid for the first time. Before taking it, he warned me to be careful of my thoughts and how they can affect me. I took the acid.

Sometime later as I was getting ready for the date, I asked him when it was going to take effect. At the time I was rubbing what I thought was some hair grease in my hands. When I looked at my hands they were black. I was about to put shoe polish in my hair! Things started happening.

On my way to pick up my date, if I thought of something sad, tears welled up quickly in my eyes. As I fought to change my sad thoughts out of fear of losing control and sobbing, the fear turn to terror. The date did not go well. On an emotional level, I was in bad shape for about a month. I never took acid again.

I described the other time earlier in the book. It was when I came back from the competency exam and entered my cell to find the illness waiting for me. I cycled rapidly between positive and negative emotions, from feeling pretty good to being paranoid. It was the first time I started thinking that something was really wrong with me.

Back to the present. As painful as it was, in the end the denial of town trips brought many gifts in the form of healing from right understanding. Right understanding equals freedom and also brings a true feeling of inner peace. The only reason the understanding and realizations came about is because I had finally reached a point in my recovery where I had become mentally and emotionally strong enough to withstand the final layer of unresolved pain without projecting it onto others. That hidden part that had been full of shame for many years was now ready to emerge from that dark, gloomy self-built prison cell. It was like stepping out into the healing rays of the sun and fresh air. I no longer needed my illness to insulate and protect me from the pain.

As a child there was no way that I could bear all that hurtful pain. The hurt felt like death. The fear of the pain had me suppressing it as best as I could. Then I had to learn to suppress the fear that also felt like death. Then I had to learn to suppress the overwhelming anger that protected me from the pain and fear. And because of the many years of suppressing it all, I became mentally ill as an adult and created destructive delusions that ended up devastating others and me. It had become far easier to create a delusion than to experience my toxic emotions.

Through the years I have been learning that real power is not about having control over others or the outcome of a situation. It's about having control over me (my thoughts, emotions, and actions) in spite of what others say or do or don't do or any other situation. I think often of something I read that stated that power over others is weakness disguised as strength and that true power is within.

This whole experience, on the clearest level ever, once again brought me back to where it all began with my family. Seeking approval for town trips was still like seeking approval from my family. I've been here almost a quarter of a century. How could this place not in some way become an extension of my family? I had come full circle.

The town trip denial brought another huge unexpected gift. Something had changed in me. I felt the change but at first there were no words to describe this change. After contemplating this for several days, I began to realize that a part of me (the little kid), no longer felt that insatiable urge and restless desire to please my parents or others any longer. I had reached a more adult place with a more appropriate level of self-esteem. It's not that I want to displease anyone; it's just that that's no longer such a strong outside drive.

Trying to please had become a hellish way of living my life. I clearly cared about others. I recognized that true caring, which is a natural part of who we are, is helping another when you can with no other reason than to just be helpful. My true caring had become contaminated, hijacked, and entangled with the desire to please and feel accepted by others. The time has come for me to fully accept myself.

It appears that this inner war that I have been fighting for over sixty years involving my unresolved emotions, that insatiable urgent desire to please my parents and others is over. Just like everyone else in this world, I want to experience the joy that comes from inner peace. A healthy separation is now taking place between pleasing and truly caring. I anticipate that this will be an adjustment that will take some time to get used to. I think the word to describe this change, the word that I had trouble finding before, is *growth*. Growth may seem like a small concept to some but for me it's huge. It's a life-affirming word. The entire experience of dealing with the possibility of town trips and then the denial of town trips caused me to reflect on and recognize a part of who I am that I hadn't thought about before.

Because of the denial of town trips, the gift I was given was to be brought face to face with my demons (toxic pain, fear, and anger). I was given the opportunity to put into practice to the fullest the taking of full responsibility for my thoughts, feelings, and actions. Because of the years of that practice, my blaming others ended much quicker than in the past, quieting those painful negative emotions to a whisper. This quieting of emotions allowed me to more clearly see not only where it all came from but also see a more constructive way of dealing with the denial of town trips.

I had a number of options for dealing with the denial. We have here a department called Patients' Rights. I can file a grievance through Patients' Rights and see if my rights were violated in any way. We have law books that I can look through for myself. When I last went to court two years ago, the last sentence in the recommendation of one of the evaluators said, "I believe that his treatment within the institution should involve a concerted effort to attempt to move Mr. Keyes to the least restrictive setting in the immediate future."

I have decided to petition the courts for release again. That same evaluator will represent me. I hope the judge will have questions about why there are unusual rules for me despite my good record and about why I haven't been transferred. Mostly, I can either continue to be thankful for all that I presently have or go on hurting and continue the vicious cycle of acting out and justifying it by blaming others. I have a strong sense that I have come full circle because of working to understand these significant events. I came back to the place of non-illness.

I now have the courage and strength to look at pain, fear, and anger as signs or guideposts letting me know that there is something I need to look at more closely. They say feelings are not bad or good, negative or positive. They are just feelings. How I choose to look at my feelings is what makes them bad or good, negative or positive. Because I feared my emotions and avoided and suppressed them through many years, it made the healing process very painful. I had to work through the emotions I was trying to hide from by experiencing them. Only by experiencing those emotions (the boogieman) without acting out did I start learning that I didn't have to fear them.

The healing process is not all painful gut-wrenching work, so don't let it scare you off! The positive parts are things like exercising, eating healthy, enjoying a hobby, spirituality, keeping good company with positive and encouraging people, and experiencing the excitement of watching my confidence grow through the years as my persistence and determination little by little overcame the illness and those things I had feared all my life.

Chapter 8

Nuts and Bolts

Here's a paraphrase of something I read once. "Evil acting people are good people who have been tortured." If I had to choose one word that helped me to work through the tortured part of me, that word would be *forgiveness*. I'll talk more about forgiveness later in this chapter.

One-on-one therapy has been great. In the beginning, having someone listen to all my craziness without judging me was like a dream come true. Still I spent days afterwards feeling vulnerable and nervous as though something was going to happen. By the next session, I was ready to continue and the same combination of awesome conversation and uncomfortable aftermath took place. Over time the uncomfortable feeling decreased. Talking about my thoughts and feelings, putting them into the light by telling them to someone else who heard them without a judgmental attitude, weakened the power the crazy thoughts and feelings had over me. It was magical and showed the healing power that comes from talking about the fears, hurts, and anger.

The trauma group was also important to my recovery. Trauma group was difficult because it involved talking about and reliving my unresolved traumatic experiences, which took having trust in others. Trust was not something I was good at, at that time.

I cannot overstate the importance of therapy to my recovery, but without paying attention to Food, Exercise, Relationships, Music, and Meditation, I don't think the therapy would have been as beneficial. The role they played in my overall recovery was and is indispensable.

Food

Just like it's said about a car, if you put bad fuel into it, it will not perform at its best. My body is no different. I have found that foods rich in nutrition or lack of it affect my energy level, which in turn can affect my attitude one way or the other. There was once an article in the local newspaper that listed foods that made you happy and foods that made you sad.

Nutritional foods give me the mental strength and staying power to deal with and work through those stressful emotional issues that were a key part of my illness. When it came to dealing with recovery issues, those unresolved issues from my past, the stresses at times were horrendous. The healthy foods had a more calming effect on me. The unhealthy foods made me more nervous and gave me an unsettled feeling.

During those times when feeling emotionally stressed, I overate and chose foods that lacked nutrition. I craved sweets, salt, and foods that left me feeling heavy. Eating replaced feeling and working through my emotions. They call it emotional eating. This was an unloving and destructive way of dealing with my emotions. The way I ate lowered my energy and made things worse.

Looking back, there was so much about food that I hadn't realized. I used to think I would feel better by smoking a joint. I never did. What I needed was a good healthy meal. Food and how food works is really quite a fascinating thing.

In the end food is nothing but energy. When my energy is high, I find it extremely difficult to stay in bad moods. So why then did I sabotage the good feelings? Because I was so addicted to living with bad feelings and the belief that I was not worthy.

As I enter the twilight of my years, I am thankful that I am staying mindful of what I eat. I do not want to leave this world thinking or feeling, "I wished I had chosen the best for myself. I wish I could have found the courage to face my fears."

Besides food helping me on the physical level, on the mental and emotional levels, my food choices help me to see where and how I'm denying myself from being the best that I can be. How I eat shows me where fear is ruling my life instead of love. Fear says I'm bad and don't deserve the best life has to offer, so when it comes to eating, eat poorly. Love says you deserve the best, so eat healthy. The way I figure it, if I give myself the best, I will have my best to give to others. They say when you feel good you can do great things.

Paraphrasing something I once read, it's not the darkness that holds some of us back. It's our light that frightens us. It went on to say that this light that frightens us is our greatness. Nutritional food is full of light.

Don't get me wrong; there are some junk foods that I'll eat from time to time. The difference is, I don't eat it often and I don't eat much of it.

I've spoken with people who believe that food is just food and that there's no difference between organic and nonorganic. I strongly believe there is. So many different pesticides have been put into our foods and there are more processed foods than ever. Unfortunately to some, greed is more important than people. There are those who will tell us things they know are not truthful just to make that buck. They don't realize that sooner or later they will suffer in some way from eating overly processed foods, too.

We don't get sick by accident or chance. If I eat poorly over a long period of time, I will eventually pay a price from eating that way.

I eat organic foods as much as I can. Whole grains like brown rice, beans, steel cut oats, multigrain or whole wheat bread, oat bran, wheat germ, and bee pollen, which is considered one of nature's perfect foods. I get the important omega-3 and other goodies from whole flax seeds that I grind up in a coffee grinder. Vegetables and fruit are also very important and full of energy. I eat very little meat because of its low energy output and the heavy feeling it gives me. I like the way one health book put it. It said if you're going to eat meat, eat it more towards the evening and come behind it with a big salad, which breaks it down more quickly. Because it takes so much energy to digest meat, that's why it suggested eating it more towards the evening. You need your energy to do your business during the day.

If I overeat on healthy foods, it will affect me negatively. The health book I read called *Fit for Life* by Harvey and Marilyn Diamond had a whole page that kept repeating, "Do not overeat!" It went on to explain the negative effects overeating has on the body, and the days it takes for your body to straighten itself out again.

One of the other things that I've noticed about not overeating and eating very lightly is that it affects my muscles as though I've been stretching. I find myself much more flexible when it comes to bending down or just plain walking. I sleep better, too.

Foods rich in nutrition are one of my most important medications. A friend who eats healthy and exercises said something really neat recently. He said, "Exercise helps distribute the nutrients throughout your body." I never thought of it in that way before. It made sense. Come to think about it, it will distribute the poor nutrients throughout my body as well.

I'll sum up food this way by saying, when eating healthy foods, the less food I eat when I eat, the more energy I experience. This way of eating makes it impossible to stay in the dumps and gives me the maximum energy and opportunity to deal with life issues.

When it comes to all these things I'm talking about—foods, exercise, relationships, and meditation—the number one enemy or hindrance has been fear. The number one liberator from all this fear has been learning what it means to love life, others, and me. "I will resist responding from a place of fear with all my heart, mind, strength, and soul. Instead, I will respond from a place of love with all my heart, mind, strength, and soul."

Exercise

Some form of exercise has been a part of my life from early childhood, but not when I was in the grip of the Force. Like food, exercise was another one of those important medication replacements that played its important role in bringing me out of my psychosis. They say exercise releases endorphins in your brain. These endorphins are said to give you a feeling of wellness and that has been my experience.

As I started healing, exercise really helped my stress level. I had to initially push through the stress and depression to do some form of exercise no matter how little it was. I might do a few stretches, something for my stomach, and something aerobic to get my heart rate up for a few minutes. It was important for me to do something in my room as I couldn't depend on someone taking me to the gym or exercise room. It was important that I didn't do too much at first so I wouldn't get discouraged and quit. Working out like I was going out for the Olympics was not going to work. And it was important to do the little I was doing on a regular basis. This helped me to stay motivated and brought some discipline into my life.

During stressful times, if I missed a few days of exercising or ate badly, as gently as I could, I reminded myself that it was okay and that I would quickly get back to doing what I knew was best for me. Over time I started adding on more and more exercises until I had a routine I didn't mind doing and that made me feel good after doing it. Just like most things you do over and over, it starts to become a habit. This was a good habit. They say repetition makes the master.

I enjoy being on the treadmill at least three times a week and sometimes more for about thirty minutes or so listening to some of my favorite music. When I'm finished, I'll be sweating all over, getting those pores cleaned out. Then I take a nice shower and just kick back or work on some project.

Presently I have a nice exercise that I do for about twenty minutes in the morning, and one that I do for about fifteen minutes in the evening involving more stretching, which helps me sleep easier instead of the tossing and turning because of tightness. I didn't realize the importance of stretching until I actually did it. I felt like I had a rebuilt body. Some of the physical pain I experienced in my legs was because of tight muscles and not necessarily old age. Once they were stretched out, the pain instantly went away until they got tight again from not stretching.

So, instead of waiting for the pain, I just stretch and if I forget, the pain will definitely remind me to do it.

Relationships

I became so used to being alone and lonely, I never gave much conscious thought to relationships. The relationships I encountered were brief and short-lived. Thoughts of relationships meant being afraid of feeling the pain of worthlessness and rejection if for some reason they decided that they didn't want to be around me anymore.

Once after living in a small community for about a year or two, I decided it was time to move on. One of the people I had gotten to know found out. When I saw her, she said, "So you're going to leave without saying anything about it?" I was dumbfounded. I couldn't believe that someone actually cared that I was leaving the area. At this moment I feel emotional just thinking about it. And that comment was made over twenty-five years ago.

My dad used to say a man was lucky if he had one friend. I had one from childhood and one I met in my early teens. Because of my restlessness and always on the move, I never spent much time with these friends as an adult. I was too busy running from the feeling of worthlessness. I was too busy running from something that was impossible to run from—myself. I think about the book by Jon Kabat-Zinn called, *Wherever You Go There You Are*.

Closer intimacy was totally out of the question. The very thought frightened me. Because of my low self-esteem, the thought of trying to be an equal partner in a relationship made me feel too dependent on another. Understanding my childhood experiences helps me to understand why close relationships have always been uncomfortable for me.

One defining childhood experience affected all relationships, intimate and non-intimate, in a profound way. I was around 7 years old at the time. The day was warm and sunny. It was a safe day. My two younger siblings and I ran home from school to eat lunch. My two older siblings walked slowly behind us. They had the key to the house. Mom was at work. When we younger kids got to the house, we waited for them but they were taking too long. The back door on the upper porch was usually open, and I had seen my older brother climb up one of the porch support beams to get in the house from time to time. I decided I was going to try it for the first time. Those daredevil games we played gave me courage.

I climbed up on to the railing and wrapped my arms and legs around the beam and started the climb. I felt determined, excited, and scared. A fall could mean serious injury or death. Once to the top, I had to transfer from the beam to the porch. That meant letting go with one arm and grabbing the railing while supporting myself on the beam with just one arm and both legs wrapped tightly around it. Then I had to let go of the beam completely and haul myself over the railing to the porch. Success! I made it! It felt so good that I had taken the risk and accomplished my goal.

The porch door was open and I went in, intending to go let the other kids in, but something, maybe a noise, made me look in the living room where my mom slept. My dad was there, too, and they were having sex, although I didn't understand it at the time.

I stood frozen in place staring. Dad saw me and shouted, "Get out of here and go out the way you came in!"

I felt like he had put a knife through my heart. I was confused, frightened, and hurt. I didn't understand what was going on and my own father was sending me back into danger.

Making it safely down the beam, I waited on the steps with my two younger sisters for someone to come and open the door. I didn't say word one about what had just happened. Mom came in her robe and let us in. We sat silently at the table while she prepared us some lunch. I don't even remember the older kids coming in. I just sat there feeling so hurt. Mom asked me a question about something related to lunch. She asked me with unusual gentleness. Her gentleness was a cool drink of water on a hot scorching day. I badly needed that cool drink at that moment.

The experience stayed locked away well into my adult years. I think it help explains why I didn't feel valued and how my sense of self-worth affected my ability to have healthy relationships.

Because of the nature of institutional life, healthy relationships are difficult to have in here. Besides that fact, I have had the opportunity and good fortune to meet some people in the community since being locked away and reestablish some old relationships from the past. At this time I can say I have several great friends. One of them is the person who was a little upset about me leaving the area without saying anything.

At first it was scary and I looked for reasons to run from these relationships. It was the emotional involvement that presented the greatest challenge. I hung in there though, and I'm thankful for facing my fears. I have found that one of the greatest healing powers in my recovery has been getting involved in caring relationships built on trust.

What astonished me the most and what I found difficult to accept at first was having people in my life that trust and care for me in spite of the things I've done. They trusted me when I didn't even trust myself. They had faith in me while I was still ill. I'm treated like a valued human being instead of a dangerous mentally ill person. I'm treated with dignity and respect, gentleness and kindness. Their confidence in me helped me to believe in myself and gave me hope.

What I look for in my relationships is what all healthy people want. They want trust, integrity, respect, and thoughtfulness. They want people who sincerely care about others.

What I know now more than ever is what it's like to be a human being. To be a human being is to recognize and not be afraid to feel my good emotions, too. Emotions like love, compassion, and gratitude make you strong rather than weak. It's also important not to fear sadness and grief.

Although I haven't found that one special person yet, I know I'm ready now for the right one. Maybe it will still happen.

I do expect to get out one day. If I'm wrong and I never see physical freedom again, there is one other relationship that can never be taken from me.

The highest and most important relationship I'll ever have is with me and the loving spirit within me. If I was not me, and I read that last statement, I would wonder where in the world was this all-loving spirit when Louie committed those horrible crimes. My answer would be that in the end, everything came down to the power of choice, right and wrong, which I lacked the capacity to have at the time. My thoughts were consumed with continuous fear, pain, and suffering. Out of sheer desperation to find meaning and purpose in my life, my reality became more and more twisted. I started seeing myself as this so-called good guy whose job it was to get rid of the so-called bad guys.

So in my last ditch effort and only after being arrested, put in a mental institution, and under the threat of being on medication for the rest of my life (which I deeply feared being controlled and dependent on) did that same feeling of desperation eventually arise again. Only this time the desperation helped me to begin self-discovery, bringing healing and the realization that I always had a choice. My past choices were based in fear, anger, worthlessness, and ignorance, which blocked the awareness of an all-loving spirit that had always been within me. I now know without a doubt that it is there. My job is to nourish it every day by being aware of it, letting it guide me, and being ever so thankful for it. The most important trust is being able to trust my values, my word, and myself. I have to earn trust, and I'm learning the ways in which I can and cannot trust others (see my poem on trust in the Songs and Poems section near the end).

Music

In spite of the terror I experienced in early childhood, in spite of the worthlessness I felt early on and through most of my adult life, through all my perceived failures in my life, one of my saving graces has been my passion for music.

Through the childhood pain, those moments of listening to the beautiful music on the radio transported me to a safe place and set me free to feel joy for a little while. Those songs carried me through as a teenager fighting through the confusion and searching for an identity. As an adult, music again carried me through as I searched desperately for my place here on earth, completely losing myself and inflicting great pain and suffering into the lives of others. And although I was looking for a gentle way to die, once again music helped see me through.

One of the most awesome feelings in the world is bringing to life a musical composition stirring in your thoughts. From its beginning to its end it's an exciting journey. It can feel like

Christmas and Santa just left. You record the part you're hearing in your soul over and over however long it takes until your heart explodes with a joy that says, "Yea! That's it!" You lay back with great satisfaction listening to it again and again. The other part that's so exciting is the thought that how can this not bring joy to someone else as well?

Speaking about Santa, I was in a group once called Dealing with Mental Illness. The facilitator asked us who would we like to be, fiction or nonfiction, and why? Some of my peers laughed when I said Santa Claus. I can understand that. Anyway, I chose Santa because he lives to just give, and how can you not be happy with a job like that? It's not about fame, power, or money.

The creation of a song can start from lyrics, a beat, or a rhythm that pops up into your head. Or melody that magically appears out of seemingly nowhere. Once I was between sleep and being awake. A melody kept going around and around in my head. It was about 3:00 in the morning. I was tired and feeling sluggish. I lay there not wanting to move but the melody persisted.

Understanding that I had to get up, I forced myself out of bed and moved awkwardly to the keyboard. I became fully awake once I started looking for the melody and its notes. I turned the drum machine on and started listening for a drum pattern that fit the melody I was hearing. Almost immediately I heard the right beat. The patterns are labeled like rock, hard rock, jazz, R&B, and so on. It was dark so I had no idea which pattern it fell under. All I know is that the drum pattern fit the melody perfect.

The sense I got from the melody and beat was that this song was for the young people that were in gangs. That excited me even more. Once the idea was completed, I became curious about the name of the pattern because it was one I wasn't used to hearing or using. To my surprise it fell under the rap category. My working song title *Believing It*, and the chorus line goes, "There's a better way my brothers and sisters, the secret is believing it." As I just reread the chorus line, I chuckled. I like that part.

Although music has been off and on for me throughout my life, finally (better late than never and right on time) I'm at a place where I know how I would like to spend my remaining days on earth. Doing music, music, and music, the universal language.

They say you can't enter this kingdom called heaven until you become childlike again. When I am creating, the child in me is alive and full of incredible joy. My love for music brought me through many of life's storms.

In order to record music here in the institution, I had to apply for what they call a patient-run business. You have to be on a certain level to get and maintain the business. To make a long story short, I got myself into some trouble and lost the business. The equipment I used to create the music was put in storage. I figured once I got my level back I could have the business back. After about a year I received a letter from security saying I had to send the equipment out because they could not be responsible if something was stolen. I was crushed.

Over time, but vague at first, I started sensing that this was an opportunity. I started seeing my dependency on music as my main source of joy, identity, and self-worth. That did not feel safe or right to me. When the equipment was taken, that death-like pain I felt when it had to be sent out showed me that. Something died in me and it had to die for something new that was waiting to be born.

As I worked through my anger and disappointment, I started to work on this memoir. The more I worked on it, the more excited I became with it. If I still had the music, I would not have put this type of energy into the memoir. Like music this memoir is a creation coming from me. And like music, I have moments of excitement about it helping others. I have discovered another possible talent. I can write. I have another way to express my thoughts and emotions creatively. And it didn't stop there.

Not having the business has given me ideas on how to use karaoke music in a creative way for making income in the future or just plain enjoying it. In fact, there's a chance I would not have even gotten into karaoke if I still had the business. All my eggs are no longer in one basket. Although very painful, everything that happened was an opportunity in disguise.

Earlier in this memoir, I mentioned the first song I wrote called, *Who Am I*. Both the earlier and a new version of the song are in the section near the end called Songs and Poems.

Relationships

I will make an attempt to share with you the most important human-to-human relationships outside of my mother that I ever had related to recovery. I shared it with you earlier. It was with The Neighborhood House and Blondie at the age of 5 and 6.

Looking back, as dark as those times were for me, it's as if my recovery was set in motion during that period of my life. The experience of that dual relationship of The Neighborhood House and Blondie instilled in me and brought to life the love and hope I would need to make it through the storms that were to come.

I truly believe and I will go as far as saying, I "know" that it was my Higher Power's way of letting me know in the most gentle, loving, and powerful way that there was something in me that was loveable in spite of the agony in my life. That magical, wonderful experience of long ago with The Neighborhood House and Blondie was the very slow beginning of my awakening (see my poem *Little Did I Know*).

Blondie was a real physical person that I met at The Neighborhood House just like I told you. And I did find her again but not physically. I found her in my spirit heart. I found her within. She never came and she never left. She was always here and was that part in me and in all of us that is pure, perfect, and divine (our innocence).

Meditation

Meditation is about going within. You hear some people say they just can't meditate. I once read something interesting about meditation. It said you couldn't drive a car or eat if you couldn't meditate. That told me that meditation is ultimately about focus and where I put my attention. If my attention is focused on negative thoughts, that means I'm thinking about or meditating on negativity. It would be the same about positive thoughts or anything else as far as that goes.

When I first started meditating I found it uncomfortable going within but that discomfort was just a smoke screen keeping me away from the good stuff, because the deeper you go within the better it gets. It's similar to digging a well for lifesaving water. The deeper you go, the tougher the ground gets. And because you didn't give up, you finally hit pay dirt. Well, actually you hit water!

What makes the difference is what I choose to meditate on. There are different types of meditations. Some people like visualizations. They might imagine themselves on a white sandy beach looking out in deep blue waters or in a quiet forest.

I started meditating after being incarcerated. Meditation has become my number one medication. The discovery of meditation has been the foundation of my recovery because of what it has done and continues to do for me. It brings clarity of mind, allowing me to effectively deal with everyday problems and adversities. Meditation moves me through and beyond my fears. When meditating, answers and solutions to problems very gently appear.

Meditation is the powerful glue that brings my life together and helps me to make sense of everyday living. This clarity allows me to see what is important, like the health of this temporal shell called a body. It helps me to make better food choices, to stay with my exercising, to value and stay committed to relationships, and to remain open to others. It enhances my energy and strengthens my will.

If I wake up in the middle of the night or can't sleep because I'm been ruminating and I'm upset about an injustice, I meditate. At a time like that, it can be very difficult to meditate. In fact, because the meditation is so opposite of what I'm used to doing when I get angry, the anger actually increases. Meditating when feeling disturbed can be like riding a bucking horse. You have to hold on. Just like digging that well, if I stay with it, mediation will eventually take me to a calmer more peaceful place.

I prefer focusing on my breath going in and out very gently, sometimes focusing on the sound OM as I breathe in and out or silently repeating an affirmation or mantra (something positive or uplifting that is repeated over and over). My purpose of meditating is primarily to get in touch with the calmer more peaceful part of me that is eternal love that I now know dwells within us all. I also believe this eternal love, this particular part within us and within me, is pure, perfect, and divine. I know it may be hard for people reading this to reconcile this belief with the horrible things I did. I can hear people saying, "How dare you?" It was hard for me, too, and some days it's still hard. My answer is, "How dare I not make a statement like that after what I've done?"

Because of early childhood experiences and teachings, I've been quick to believe in my sense of worthlessness and that has brought nothing but pain and suffering. So it makes sense to me to undo that old teaching by practicing and believing in the eternal love within.

When I first started meditating, my stress—created by my fear and worry—did become more noticeable and distinct. The fear and troublesome thoughts kept going around and around in my mind. It was uncomfortable and even a little scary at times. I wanted to give up, but I learned to continue breathing in and out focusing on my breath as best as I could. When my attention went to my thoughts, I gently brought the focus back to my breath. It was only because of my determination to heal and be the best person I could that I stayed with it. Plus I knew the other worthless alternative all too well.

The most challenging thing I find about meditating on inner love is that anything that isn't part of this love and anything that blocks the experience of this love reveals itself. Feelings of fear, hate, negativity, and worthlessness rise to the surface and compete with the growing awareness of your inner love.

Let's say I'm meditating on the affirmation, "I'm pure, perfect, and divine," or "We are all pure, perfect, and divine." This pure, perfect, and divine part is called by many names, such as the Holy Spirit, the Great Spirit, the Source, and chi. In the beginning because of old conditioning, I could hardly think the words I'm pure, perfect, and divine let alone say them. It's very difficult to change or see yourself differently when you believe and have been told over, and over, and over, and over again, and again, and again, that you are a sinner! After a while no one had to tell me that I was a sinner any more. I learned to do it all by myself. I bought in to believing I was a sinner and worthless. And I kept confirming it through my negative thinking and actions. I became my biggest enemy.

Committing a sin does not make me a sin, does it? I once read something that said that one of the biggest sins a person can commit is not loving others or oneself and seeing oneself as worthless.

This is one of my challenges. Upon saying that I'm pure, perfect, and divine, my inner war starts up because of my old sinner conditioning. The blockade that's keeping me from the experiences of the inner love reminds me that I'm worthless. Back and forth the warring dialogue rages: "I'm pure," "I'm worthless," "I'm a sinner," "I'm pure," "I'm worthless," "I'm a sinner."

I find meditating on the pure, perfect, and divine affirmation very difficult because of those many years I spent thinking and feeling that worthlessness. So sometimes I go back to something that was also challenging at the start like, "I'm a good person." But I don't give up on pure, perfect, and divine. I keep chipping away at it every chance I get.

I remember a peer saying or doing something that was very hurtful and it really made me angry. I immediately started saying, "I'm pure, perfect, and divine" over and over and simultaneously felt the sense of hurt and worthlessness trying to take me over as my anger and my determination to get through this intensified. After some time of staying with it, the tears started streaming down my face and I said the words, "Thank you." The tears were the sign letting me know that on this occasion I broke through the pain of worthlessness. The poison of this portion of worthlessness was being purged through the tears. It took far more courage, strength, and I might say hard work to cry than to hurt someone. Later on I could say of the peer, "He's pure, perfect, and divine."

Tears are not just about feeling the hurt. Nor are they solely about the cleansing of emotions. Tears helped me feel empathy for myself and feeling empathy for myself in turn led me to shedding tears and feeling empathy for the suffering of others. As my fear lessened, it was replaced by growing empathy for my peers, the staff, friends, family, and those who I see on the news who have lost a loved one or whose home was destroyed by a natural disaster. I feel deep sadness when I think of the plight of the Syrian refugees and those who can't get out and the children who live with bombs falling, little water and food, and no place to play. This is a change for me.

Since coming to this institution I've gotten back the feeling for others' suffering that I had as a kid and as a teen. I don't know when I lost it. I didn't even know it was gone until it started coming back. I think that meditation, tears, merging with the light within, and empathy for self creates emotional and spiritual strength. Then the practice of meditation deepens that strength, and empathy for others is one of the flowers that grows from this strong root structure.

So now I am experiencing a brand new toughness—it's the toughness to be human, to feel my emotions, and to express them in an appropriate way. The shame and the guilt and the sorrow over a past that I cannot change remain—they are part of who I am—but as a backdrop allowing me to see the good that I can do in the present.

Over time I have been slowly reaping the rewards of being persistent with meditating. I'm having more clarity and less confusion, fear, and worry. The troublesome thoughts are starting to fade more to the background as the healthy part of me is naturally surfacing on its own.

They say you should burn up your impurities (negativity) in the fire of meditation. To me this means, when meditating, I should keep focusing on my breath slowly going in and out, in and out, in and out. To burn up means to dissipate or become irrelevant over time. Even if some of the negativity sneaks back in (and it more than likely will!), it will not have its old impact.

I must say there have been times when something would come up that was very painful and I felt like I hadn't gotten anywhere with meditation. The truth was that I indeed did get somewhere. This was just some more old unresolved stuff that I was ready for and needed to work through.

One of the other neat things about meditation is I can do it anytime, anywhere. I can be standing in line. I can choose to do it instead of getting caught up in anger or some other kind of negative emotion. If I was stuck in traffic I could meditate. The point is not for me to meditate only when a problem comes up but to do it on a regular basis. Then it acts like a protective shield. It's like saving money in a bank for when I need it. Meditation is security.

Spirituality

Back to the pure, perfect, and divine mantra. If there is a God, Higher Power, or whatever you call God, and this God is pure, perfect, and divine, and loves us all unconditionally, to me it makes sense that there must be something in us and in me that is also pure, perfect, and divine and that God finds worth loving. Nothing else makes sense to me. God knows we are much more than our mistakes and impurities.

In thinking about the part in the Bible where Jesus says, *the kingdom of God is within you,* I contemplated what that meant for me. One thing for sure, it can mean different things for different people at different times in their lives as they journey through this life. I believe none of us are necessarily right or wrong. In the end things fit where they fit for us as individuals and if the fit is not right, I believe it will straighten itself out on its own time.

Let me put it this way. Like you, I am not perfect. My body has a beginning and an end. I don't believe this body is the kingdom. It's the spirit within that animates this body that is the kingdom. And it is this spirit within us, within me that is pure, perfect, and divine. I believe the more one believes and meditates or contemplates this spirit, the more one merges with it.

Therefore, one begins to experience that peace that is also spoken about that goes beyond one's understanding. It's not about a knowing or a head thing, but more about that experience. I've had the habit of trusting my doubting mind rather than the positive experiences. You heard that saying about renew your mind by renewing your thoughts? It can be easier said than done but if I truly want peace, it has to be done. My fear based thoughts eventually led to a severe mental illness. No renewal; no peace. I'm not saying I'm right. They're just my thoughts and what I've been experiencing up to this point in my life.

Further proof for me of the strong possibility of the pure, perfect, and divine part in us came again as I was sitting in my room one day. Out of nowhere I started feeling a kind of mild euphoric feeling. Since I wasn't on any medication I started wondering if they slipped some in my food. Keep in mind this happened over twenty years ago. Anyway as I was trying to figure out why I was feeling so good, I thought if it was a drug it didn't feel like one. And I surely wasn't used to feeling that way.

I continued to ponder why this good feeling was happening. I started picturing in my mind the different ladies I knew in my life.

Surely it had to be one of them I was unconsciously thinking about on some level. People just don't feel good for no reason, do they? Then I caught myself and thought, "Will you look at me looking for a reason to justify this feeling instead of accepting it as possibly being the natural state of well-being, which is our true selves, my true self."

The bottom line is this, people will move in the direction of their predominate thoughts. If their predominate thoughts are about their worthlessness and they believe it, they will without a doubt, consciously or unconsciously think in ways and act in ways to make that worthless belief a reality. As far as I'm concerned—been there and done that.

They say the proof is in the pudding. For me it's very simple. There is no way that my desire and determination alone, although they helped, could have overcome the severity of my illness. Believing in a love within me that was greater than my illness or any problem was one of the secrets to overcoming it.

How can I give the best of my best if I don't think on the best or feel my best? I believe in a Higher Power. I believe the greatest honor I can give this power is to learn to love others and me like the Higher Power loves us, loves me.

I heard the spiritual teacher Dr. Wayne W. Dyer once quote Pierre Teilhard de Chardin, SJ. "We are not human beings having a spiritual experience. We are spiritual beings having a human experience." I really like that a lot. It helped me change the way I looked at my fellow human beings.

My new path is to go in the direction of believing that there's a part in all of us that is pure, perfect, and divine. This way of thinking makes my life far more exciting. Plus, it helps me to look for the best in others.

I read another statement many years ago. Through the years I think of it from time to time. Over time this statement has been becoming more and more understandable. The statement went something like this, "The deeper the pain and sorrow a person endures, the greater capacity they have for joy and love." This explains the joy and love I am experiencing more and more. All adversities, as difficult and painful as they may be, can be viewed as opportunities to transform my thinking. There are many moments that I feel such gratitude that the tears just come flowing down. They say your thoughts create your feelings, and your feelings can magnify your thoughts. (Read the poems called "Thinking" and "I Choose Love" in the Songs and Poems section near the end.)

Chapter 9

Conclusion

There's a very big difference between someone with mental illness who has committed a crime and someone who hasn't. I was listening to a radio program and the speaker talked about how when someone has done something wrong, you never know if they're going to do it again. It really brought home the legitimate concerns folks have about those of us who have committed serious crimes. It helped me better understand the additional fears people have about those of us with mental illnesses who want to work on our recovery without medication. Each person has to find a way to prove they have recovered and that they have learned the skills to lead a healthy and sane life. Some people will never believe you can recover, and some will give you a chance. Even without a mental illness, some people will never believe someone who committed a crime can be a decent and productive member of the community.

Suffering

When suffering "from" something, there's more of a tendency to repress the hurt or act upon the hurt which leads to a continuous recycling of the suffering. And so you're trapped in the suffering. When suffering "through" something, the healing comes when I feel the pain, fear, or anger without avoiding it and without acting upon it.

Medication

Like I said, I am not anti-medication. There's no doubt in my mind that medication can play a very important role in recovery. It can help stabilize someone who is going through a crisis. After the crisis is over, I think it's important to help that person to find their voice and give them all the known facts so they can make an informed decision regarding how they would like to use or not to use medication.

My medication is a different sort of medication. I consider nutritional foods and exercise as my medication of choice. My medication is also having a purpose. Having purpose inspires me daily. My medication is the people who treat me with dignity, respect, kindness, and understanding. I love being around people who are encouraging and positive, and so I seek them out. I already know how to be negative; I had great examples of that growing up. I don't like being that way. My medication is mindfulness. I am continually learning to watch my thoughts and replace the negative ones with positive ones—I love affirmations—and I'm learning to be aware of my negative thoughts without getting caught up in them. My medication is learning to forgive others and myself.

If some people had their way, the whole world would be on medication. If you doubt this, read the book called *Anatomy of an Epidemic: Magic Bullets, Psychiatric Drugs, and the Astonishing Rise of Mental Illness in America* (2010) by Robert Whitaker. If you think that people can never recover and become medication-free, watch a DVD called *Take These Broken Wings* (2008). It's a documentary by Daniel Mackler on two individuals who were diagnosed with severe schizophrenia and are medication-free. One of those two people is Joanne Greenberg. She's the author of *I Never Promised You a Rose Garden* (1964). A friend who recently saw *Take These Broken Wings* said the information is irrefutable. Another interesting DVD documentary also by Daniel Mackler is *Open Dialogue* (2011) about an innovative relational, non-anti-psychotic medication approach to schizophrenia based in Finland. Finland has the best statistical results in the world for first-break psychosis. They have an 85 percent recovery rate, medication-free.

Whitaker and Mackler cared enough to seek the truth and share it with us. They display the type of courage that is in all of us if we will only take hold of it. They show us what it means to truly care about others and also how to open their minds to other ways and other ideas. By making this invaluable information available, with this knowledge, I now have a responsibility to share it when appropriate opportunities arise. I pray for the wisdom to know when and how to share it.

Someone once said that there are people who have recovered and don't know it. My first thought was how is this possible? The person gave a true life example of someone, who I will call Bob, who thought he was still mentally ill because he still felt anger. Of course people who aren't mentally ill feel anger so why does Bob think he is mentally ill because he still feels anger?

Bob doesn't have the information he needs to make an informed assessment about his mental health. If I have that information, is it my responsibility to share the information with him? Where does my responsibility stop and start? How much responsibility does Bob have to seek out information?

It's different in each situation. One thing I do know, however, is that in sharing information, there are big pieces, little pieces, and little tiny pieces, but there's no such thing as an insignificant piece. Each piece of information about mental health and mental illness is critical to the success of the whole. As far as I'm concerned, the most difficult piece, the big piece, was already accomplished when Whitaker and Mackler published the book and produced the DVDs.

As far as a little piece goes, let's say I've been telling people they will have to be on medication for the rest of their lives so get used to it. After reading the Whitaker and Mackler book and watching the DVDs, I have new information and I can decide to tell or not to tell this new information to people. If I want people to share in their own healthcare decisions, I will decide to tell them the whole story. Then if they do end up on medication for the rest of their lives, it won't be because in their most vulnerable moment I told them only one piece of the story and told them as if that piece was true and inevitable when an alternative medical protocol that is equally true and fact-based is successfully practiced in other communities. I am living proof that the medication route is not the only possible effective route.

Again, a little tiny piece is just as important as the big piece. I might be looking at someone or a group of people or just thinking about people and say to myself something like, "I wish them joy, peace, and the healing they need in their lives." I have learned that thoughts are very powerful. Thoughts have energy.

I made very few allies in my quest to be medication-free, but the few I did make had a tremendous influence on me. In so many ways it was like me in conflict with the whole institution. Then I discovered the National Empowerment Center out of Lawrence, Massachusetts. One of the founders is a courageous man named Daniel Fisher. In his twenties he was diagnosed with schizophrenia. Daniel told his treating doctor at the time that he wanted to become a psychiatrist. Instead of Daniel's doctor thinking of him as being grandiose as some surely might, the doctor told Daniel that he wanted to attend his graduation. Daniel went on to get his doctorate in psychiatry at Harvard University. Daniel's doctor believing in him helped give him the courage and confidence to believe in himself. He went on to get his doctorate in biochemistry at the University of Wisconsin.

Volunteers run the National Empowerment Center. They are great people who have been there and done that! For me, it was like finding a family who truly understood. They have a wealth of information for anyone serious about recovery. Every mental institution in the country should be knocking down their door for that wealth of information. How fortunate I am to have discovered them. I can hardly keep the smile off my face just writing this. So, I'll just smile. Thank you, Empowerment Center!

Unlike in other countries, in our country's mental illness system it is considered unusual or impossible for a person to recover from a mental illness like schizophrenia. It's considered even more impossible to recover while remaining medication-free. At the institution where I live, a chart is kept in a binder and contains each patient's personal information. Staff members write in the chart daily to describe negative or positive events that occur. Clinicians write in it about once a month and give an overview of that month. Keeping in mind that I've been here over 25 years, a new clinician recently charted the following opinion.

> Again, there has been the question as to whether he ever really had a primary psychotic disorder, as it is unusual to have had a complete resolution of symptoms with no recurrence without any sort of ongoing medication treatment.

The clinician who wrote this was not here in the beginning to witness my severe state, nor to watch the struggles and hard work I've put in to get to this point while remaining medication-free. I definitely felt some frustration but kept in mind the understanding that this clinician received a Western education and was taught the Western medical model of mental illness and mental health. The clinician who questioned whether I ever really had a psychotic disorder must not trust his peers' clinical abilities to give an accurate diagnosis. Before being sentenced here, two prominent psychiatrists, one who represented the prosecution, diagnosed me as having Acute Paranoid Schizophrenia. Others here besides the new clinician have also questioned my recovery. Of course, if someone only has a limited experience and is not used to seeing something, how can I really knock them for their disbelief? Their skepticism is understandable. I remember reading in Whitaker's book *Anatomy of an Epidemic* that most clinicians never hear about the many who are successful and who go on to lead productive lives without medication. They just keep seeing the many who keep returning. So if you think about it that way, it makes sense that it can be a hard sell to convince clinicians and staff members that mental illness is an illness like any other and recovery is possible like with other illness.

I am by no means saying that knowing this information and broadening our understanding of mental illness and recovery is enough on which to base a decision to release me or anyone back into the community. Recognizing that medication-free recovery is possible and that alternatives to medication are being successfully practiced opens a different kind of door. I can only think that fewer limits on treatment possibilities might mean a better chance of finding a treatment match for more individuals suffering from schizophrenia.

I recovered by slowly piecing together a daily regimen and life plan that works for me. Even though I recovered medication-free, I recovered with the help of the many talented clinicians and kind people and resources that the institution placed at my disposal and encouraged me to use. I mean, it all worked. Why is it that once successful, some of the very people who gave me the mental health tools then doubted I was ever mentally ill or think the original diagnosis must have been wrong. Instead, shouldn't they be saying, "Every person's victory is our victory, too?" Now, that would be a truly awesome day.

Caregivers

To those who work with the mentally ill, especially the aides that work the most directly with us on a daily basis, you play a most important role in our recovery. You have great and probably unsuspected power over how our days shape up, what we think about our self-worth, and our next steps on our road to mental health.

I believe that most caregivers have no idea of the power of their words, gestures, facial expressions, tone, body language, and actions. We, the mentally ill, are in some ways as defenseless as newborn babies in the beginning of our recovery process. How we're treated by you at that time greatly impacts our lives. Further into the recovery process, these things have far less of an impact on us. This is why especially in the beginning it is imperative that you understand your significance and power and treat us with great, great care and thoughtfulness.

Let's say a caregiver has a rough night in some way. Maybe he or she was up most the night with a sick child. That person may come to work tired and snappish because of something that has absolutely nothing to do with those in his or her charge. When those who are mentally ill are not very far on their journey to health, a caregiver's angry tone can easily send the patient into a tailspin filled with anguish.

I remember once early in my journey to recovery I approached the nursing station to ask for something and was met with a harsh response. Back then it was easy for me to think they didn't like me and had something against me. I would think they were out to get me and hurt me in some way. The next day they could be having an innocent conversation with another caregiver about a car accident they witnessed coming in to work that morning, and I overhear it. I would think they were threatening to run over me or someone I cared for with their car if they ever got the chance. The caregiver would not have a clue that this was going on in my mind.

Recently, in fact just the other day, a caregiver I never saw before was in the nurse's station with the request window closed.

She appeared tired because her eyes kept opening and closing. By some of her expressions she looked like this was not the place she wanted to be. The request window is usually opened by 7:30 a.m. When 7:30 came I knocked on the door. She gave me the most annoyed glance I had ever seen since being here. If looks could kill, I didn't stand a chance. I thought to myself, "Wow!" She probably had no idea how she was coming across. I thought about how devastating that look would have been early on in my recovery. It could have not only played a part in wrecking my day but also a part in wrecking my week, month, yes, and even year. I promise you, there are no exaggerations here. This is serious stuff.

If caregivers truly understood this power they have, they would either be excited with enthusiasm in knowing the great contribution they can make to a life or not want to work here because of the tremendous responsibility.

Caregivers please understand your power and influence. You have the potential to play a very significant part in our success. Try to make it a point regardless of how you might be feeling on any given day to come to work and leave work knowing you did your very best that day to be kind. Like most things, the more and longer you practice something the better you get at it. You don't have to have all the answers. Just be gentle, kind, thoughtful, and willing to listen. There's no better therapy for you or for us. It wasn't until later on my road to mental health that I could understand that you, too, have struggles in life.

Lack of Knowledge

All of us are living with various degrees of ignorance. Sometimes it takes the most painful experiences to wake us up from that sleep of ignorance.

In dealing with the staff and my peers related to my recovery, it has been like going through a complex and difficult obstacle course. There is never, and I mean never a dull moment. They all have played an essential part in my healing. It was those staff people who were gentle and treated me with dignity and respect that made the greatest impact in my recovery. They gave me hope and the confidence that I could recover. I must say that some of the gentleness I received frightened me at first.

As I got healthier, those staff that brought a negative attitude to work and projected their problems onto us patients as well as their own peers also played their parts in my recovery. Just like in the real world, everyone you meet, every situation is not going to be peaches and cream. The negative staff people ended up making me stronger by giving me the opportunity to work on not taking things personally. There was nothing easy about it though. Don't get me wrong, there were many times I would wish they could be transferred to another planet. My peers gave me the opportunity to work on things like patience, control, tolerance, understanding, and how to stay away from certain people that you have to live with in close quarters daily. Dealing with institutional living is a constant test. Everything that I'm confronted with here is an opportunity for growth.

The one other thing I found to be very important in my healing process is the need to be aware of and count the very smallest of my successes in recovery. For example, I noticed that instead of being angry for one hour over a situation, I was angry for fifty-three minutes. My small successes gave me hope, encouragement, and showed me that I was making progress. I had to be determined, persistent, and patient. In doing these three things, I practiced thinking "when I recover" and not "if I recover." Whenever I fell off the horse, I didn't kick the ground and stomp away calling myself a lousy cowboy. No, I dusted off my 10-gallon hat, clapped it back on my head, and got back on the horse.

Forgiveness

I think one of the greatest teachings is, "Forgive them for they know not what they do." Forgiveness has played a crucial part in my recovery process. The difficult struggle I experienced in forgiving, in the end, was more than worth it. Forgiving others, although hard to do, seemed relatively simple compared to forgiving myself. What I realized after a while was that forgiving others was directly linked to forgiving myself. At times, *saying* I forgive someone was far easier than *feeling* the forgiveness towards them. I learned and experienced that sometimes my feelings were far more truthful than my words.

I believe I can only forgive others to the degree that I forgive myself. The same is true with love. I can only love others to the degree that I love myself.

If I truly wanted joy and peace in my life, I had to learn to forgive. One of the biggest obstacles in the way of forgiveness is people's belief that forgiving someone means the injustice that was done to them is somehow okay now or that they have to start hanging out with the person that has mistreated them. Not only is this absolutely not true, any injustice has consequences. I remember when the forgiveness group I attended first started. One of the members was so upset with the thought of forgiving those who tormented him as a child, he never came back. It was like he was holding on to his bitterness for dear life. Because of his pain, bitterness, and inability to forgive his tormentors at that point in time in his life, his suffering continued. It was so hard for him to understand that *those injustices would never be okay.*

I could relate to him. As a child, suppressing my hurts, anger, and fear was the way I learned to protect myself from experiencing those awful, painful, and frightening emotions, too. It created for me bitterness and endless suffering right on up into my adult life. I had no idea that I was projecting my pain and fear onto others and creating even more suffering for myself by not forgiving. When I chose to forgive, it was because I was so tired of suffering. I wanted joy and peace in my life.

When I was finally able to accept that, like me, my tormenters were human beings who also struggled and lived with hurts and fears, it helped me to move towards forgiving them. Not forgiving not only caused me endless suffering, it also had a negative effect on those I was around and cared for. You know what it's like to be around someone who is unhappy, especially if you care for them.

Even if someone does something on purpose to hurt me, they are doing it out of their own hurt, pain, fear, and ignorance. Because of that great reward of inner peace that has started to grow within me, the more I practice forgiveness the easier it becomes to practice it.

The glue that makes all recovery practices possible, I call spirituality. In all of us, in spite of our shortcomings, lives an unconditional loving spirit. In fact, I don't know how I could have possibly overcome the odds stacked against me if that loving spirit didn't live within me.

Wrapping Up

Because feeling worthless became my normal, undoing it is some of the hardest work I have ever done. It would have been easier just to commit suicide. In fact I had to pass through suicidal thoughts and an attempt before the veil of my ignorance began to lift and allowed me to see the truth of my life.

Even though I had extreme distrust for others during this journey, my desire to be healed pushed me through that distrust and allowed the important guidance of others to help me. My bulldog determination to recover would not have been enough had I not rediscovered my Higher Power. Not the God that I learned about as a young child that lived way up in the sky waiting to punish me for every mistake, but one whose spirit was within me, that loved me unconditionally, and was far bigger than my illness. Any illness.

So far in this book, I have not spoken of atonement. Atonement is a difficult, even excruciating, idea for me to talk about and yet the need to atone for the horrific things I did and their tragic consequences to others is very real and very present. The help I receive from others has helped me face this most challenging and painful burden in my life. This burden is learning to live for the remainder of my life with the knowledge that I took a human life—more than one—and caused tremendous pain and suffering to their loved ones and to mine. How can I possibly atone for that? I had to come to a realization that atonement and being forgiven by the people I injured is not the same thing. I can learn to live a life of atonement without receiving the forgiveness of others. In fact, understanding that very thing is part of living a life of atonement.

To me, atonement means at all times and to the best of my ability to treat every single person in a loving, caring way regardless of my own situation and state of mind. To always and continuously remind myself to remain peaceful regardless of how I feel. I'm learning to keep peace front and center by being mindful of living from *a place of peace and kindness* regardless of any stress or feelings of anxiety. Living from a place of peace and kindness the best I can brings greater patience and clarity (understanding).

One day while reading the newspaper in the dayroom, I overheard a peer, who I'll call Marty, call someone an ugly name. Marty laughed while saying this cruel thing to another. The victim also laughed and I knew the victim of the cruelty was masking incredible pain and embarrassment. I knew because several years before Marty had laughed in just that same way when I was performing at an institution talent show. I was instantly furious for the victim and for me as I remembered the earlier incident. Marty's laugh and the memory also triggered an older memory of when as a teen I was laughed at when singing and had laughed, too, to show I was part of the "joke" and to cover my hurt, even while I silently questioned my singing abilities.

That day in the dayroom, even though Marty and I had developed a casual, respectful relationship, I decided not to say anything. I was furious and I wanted to tell Marty about what he'd done and its impact, but I restrained myself. I reminded myself to live my life from a place of peace. Maybe there would never be a good opportunity to say anything to Marty, but saying something then had the potential to cause more of a problem.

The decision not to say anything gave me time to process my anger, hurt, and fear. A week or two went by and a new opportunity to talk with Marty presented itself. Now I could speak from a place of peace. I explained how his words and actions made me feel and Marty apologized. Because I could speak from a place of peace, Marty could respond from a place of peace.

Atonement is not about changing a past that cannot be changed. Atonement is not about making up for the suffering I've caused. I can't do either of those things. Living a life of atonement is about a commitment to strive at all times to be the very best person I can be. Now that the veil of mental illness has lifted, I can recognize the reality of my life. Now that I know better, it's imperative that I do better. Now that I am committed to *living* my atonement, I must strive each day, each hour, each minute to live from a place of peace.

I had a hard time figuring out and understanding that not only did I matter and was loveable, the truth is that I have always mattered and was always loveable even though I may not have acted or felt like it most times. I believe Love is the ultimate understanding and it does not hurt. If I am hurting, I eventually find out that my understanding of the situation is still in the process of developing. I also accept that we each will find the ultimate love (spiritual) in our own unique way, traveling our own unique paths, in our own right time.

Love is my birthright. It wasn't necessary for me to be anyone special. Ultimately the hell I've been waking up from has been of my own making. As the saying goes, "We make our own heaven or hell right here on earth."

I'm not saying that there were not reasons that played a part in me ending up in hell. I had to stop using those reasons as an excuse to remain in hell. I couldn't keep blaming the job I lost or didn't get or that my parents or siblings didn't love me or that I was abused. Once I started realizing the great power I possessed called free will, as difficult as it was at times, I started to choose how I was going to think about the situations I encountered in life now. Blaming others for how I felt, thought, and acted had to stop. At my present age (moving towards 70), I am under no illusions about my mortality. My life is coming to an end. I don't want to look back and say, "I wish I had found the courage to face my pain and fears." The choices I make are the doors to my liberation or my continued self-imprisonment; my heaven or hell.

Looking back over my life, I know something has been watching over me. Despite all the shortcomings and mistakes, I'm still here and I've been given the opportunity to change my life and make amends for my mistakes as best as I can. This year when so many are going through extremely difficult times because of the economic recession the world is recovering from, I understand how well I have it compared to others. I have food, health care, and a roof over my head. I have a bed, clean linen, heat for the cold nights and days, air conditioning for some of those smothering hot days of summer, clean drinking water, a shower, soap, and I can order a pizza now and then.

I might be locked up, but I'm freer than I've ever been as I continue my journey towards wholeness. I learned that true freedom comes from within and never from without. What would I do if I was ever released? I would find a quiet place where I could live simply and spend the remainder of my days writing songs.

One thing I know for sure is that if I walk out tomorrow but am not free within, *I am not free.*

I was reading an outstanding book by Bo Lozoff called we're *All Doing Time.* In it are many letters written to Bo by prisoners. In this one particular letter a prisoner shared that he was in prison for taking a life. I related to him when he said he felt the pain would never leave. Caught off guard at what he said next, my heart immediately felt the truth of his words. He said that his pain is a clear connection of love to the person whose life he took. Before that statement I never consciously thought of my pain and my remorse as a form of loving. Viewing my pain in this new context, I now whole-heartedly accept and welcome it. I should feel pain for what I did. My pain is no longer something I try to escape from; now it's a light or a beacon that plays an important part in guiding me. Experiencing pain and remorse and guilt are appropriate when we perform acts of evil or cruelty or negligence or withholding what someone else needs or simple meanness. My pain and remorse are a sign of my health. I am thankful for that prisoner as well as for all the other prisoners' letters of sharing and insights.

What would I like for you to remember the most and why? What I would like for you to remember the most is that no matter what past, present, or future mistakes are made, and no matter how badly one might think of others or oneself, inside at the very core is a spirit that is pure, perfect, and divine.

Our thoughts, plus the degree to which we believe in them, have great, great power and influence over how we will experience and deal with life's adversities (opportunities). The more we focus on that pure, perfect, and divine spirit, which is our true selves, the more we play a part in helping the world become a better place and each individual become the best person he or she can be. Unlike the human spirit, which CAN be broken, our divine spirit is incorruptible and CANNOT be broken. And there is nothing, nothing, and I mean nothing anyone can do to destroy that spirit. Because of free will, we can deny it; because of mental illness we can lose sight of it; but just like on a cloudy day, the sun is still there.

So we might as well suffer through all the crap we have been conditioned to believe about others and ourselves, rediscover that incorruptible spirit, and own it. It belongs to us all. It is a courageous process, and I can think of nothing more important in life to accomplish. You'll never know the people you'll help by embracing it. Fear is the one barrier to achieving this goal, but I have discovered that I can work to find and celebrate the spirit even when I am afraid. So can you.

Along the path to recovering and reclaiming your divine humanity, you'll find it can be very helpful when others believe in you. But in the end, believing in yourself is the greatest gift you can give to others and yourself. It is my deepest hope that you realize what you are capable of when you believe in yourself in a constructive way. As much as I'd like to keep talking about it, I'll stop here. Thank you for taking the time to read this memoir.

▲▼▲▼▲

Here is a reminder of what I consider key components to my recovery work and my continuing attention to my mental health and spiritual growth.

- Believing I could recover/determination
- Reliving experiences/without acting out
- Inner child work
- Reflection
- Purpose/reason for getting up each day
- Courage/overcoming my fears
- Affirmations
- Physical health/eating well, exercise
- Positive as well as negative staff and peers
- Kindness, wisdom, time, companionship, and financial help from family and friends
- Honesty/trust
- Remorse
- Meditation
- Forgiveness
- Atonement

And especially,

- Spirituality

Songs and Poems

DEDICATION

I can't go back no matter what I say or do.
The past can't change, no matter how much I wish it to.

I have done some things that I wish could be changed.
For so many my actions have caused them
A river of pain, pain, pain. Lives have been
Altered. They will never be the same.
And I must learn to live with and
Overcome my shame.

The anger and hate you might feel when thinking
Of the one who did this, it is understandable, in
So much pain, you lost a loved one. Pain so
Deep, you feel like you are dying. Sorrow
So deep you feel like you're never going
To stop crying.

And I can't go back, no matter what I say or do.
The past can't change, no matter how much I wish it to.
I just can't go back, no matter what I say or do.
The past can't change no matter how much I wish it to.

This river of pain it runs far. It has left an indelible scar.
This river of pain is so deep, it even visits me in my
Sleep. Victims' loved ones, and my loved ones, too,
All of us in so much pain, we're doing
Our best to work it through.

For the things I have done, nowhere to run or hide,
There is no escape. A much better life I will make,
By eliminating my self-hate. Mentally I'll
Dedicate my life to becoming a healthier
Man, and honor those who I've hurt
By helping who I can.

WHO AM I?

(First Version)

Who am I? I'm somebody. Who am I? I'm nobody.
It keeps me running and running, running and running,
Running and running – This thing inside of me
Keeps me running and running.

What is this invisible force that drives me on endlessly?
Could it be this thing they call fate, I hope and pray that
It's not hate. Where will it end? Does this happen to all men?
Who has control? Nobody knows; nobody knows.

Sometimes I feel so all alone, the emptiness hurts
but I must go on.
I'm living in death and I know not how long, the times I must die
before I reach home.

Will I make it? Won't somebody tell me, tell me, tell me please!
Will I or won't I ever succeed? Will I make it? Won't somebody
Please, please tell me now, what in the world is going to
Happen to me?

This may be something and it might be nothing.
All I know is, it's the way I feel sometimes.
Who am I?

LITTLE DID I KNOW

For the first time in my life because of you I felt loved.
And when you went away—I returned back to the darkness.
For so many years I searched everywhere to find you.
Cause through those years my heart just would not let you go.
But you were nowhere, nowhere, nowhere to be found.

Little did I know, I could never be satisfied
until I found you again.
Little did I know that the short sweet encounter we had
so long ago would see me through.

Love, you had the key that set me free.
You were the one who helped me see.

The love you gave was so simple and so sweet
a love that someone knew would cancel defeat.
Those struggles ahead unforeseen by me
would need a love so great, a love so true,
a love you knew would pull me through.

THE LIGHT

The light that light that never goes out
Is what living life is all about

The brilliancy can hardly be believed
This light you see was never conceived

The light that light, it's always there
Waiting to guide you with special care

Not by vision of the eyes
But of the heart, which is always wise

No danger can touch you, nothing should dare
Just sit back and relax in your easy chair

IT'S NOT OVER

I used to think
Because I made a mistake
My life was over
And sometimes I felt
I did not deserve to be alive
But I kept waking up
And I used to wonder why?

Each day becomes a new beginning
An opportunity for winning
Instead of just ending the days
It's a chance to start changing my ways

One's character is not built in a day
It takes time; it takes persistence
To learn to be gentle with oneself
I have to learn from within to listen

TRUST

They say all great relationships are built on trust
and the distrust you feel is understandable
I cannot change the past but I can change each moment
that comes
Hear me now, I cannot change the past but I can change
those moments that come.

This feeling of distrust I know so well
It's been my favorite companion;
Never letting anyone get too close,
I could not even trust myself.

It hurts, not to trust anything. It hurts.
A distrusting soul is a lonely way to live.
Always afraid and feeling so lost.
It was the only life I knew.
Every day became a struggle;
So hard to get through.

I realize you're going to think what you think
Feel what you feel and do what you do.
That's okay, I understand, it's about trust, isn't it? It's about trust.

I'm becoming a new man.

I'm finally learning to trust; sometimes it's not easy

But it feels good and I like it

Some of us do change; we are all not the same.

Some of us do change, will you, can you, give me a chance?

WHO AM I?

(Second Version)

Hey Dad, hey Dad, hey Dad –
There's something I want to say to you.
And I know you only did what you knew how to do.

Who am I? Am I somebody? Who am I? Am I nobody?
Who am I? Am I somebody? Who am I? Or am I nobody.

When I needed your love the most you were just like some kind
of ghost.
And on those rare occasions you came around but without a
sound.
Just once I wish you could have put your arms around me
To let me know I had some worth and that I was more than dirt.

Now many years have gone by and I'm a little older.
I'm tired of carrying all this hurt it's too much for these shoulders.
Inner freedom is all I truly want, this struggle has taken its toll
And now it's losing its hold.

I hate what you did to me but I don't hate you.
I hate what you did to me why couldn't you be a friend.
I hate what you did to me but I don't hate you.
I hate what you did to me no longer will I be blue.

Who am I? Am I somebody? Who am I? Am I nobody?

Who am I? Am I somebody? Who am I? Or am I nobody.

Now take the judge downtown, he's somebody.

What about the man he sent to jail, he's still somebody.

The rich man up the street is somebody.

The poor man that can't eat, is still somebody

Everybody, Everybody, Everybody is Somebody

Everybody, Everybody, Everybody is Somebody

AM I? I AM!

Am I worthy? Are you worthy too?
    And are we all worthy? If not what must I do?
        Searching everywhere just to find where I belong.
        Loneliness is not; it's not my true home.

Money, fame, neither will do, to win life's game
    I must, I must find you, where? Within
        Am I worthy? Are you worthy too?

Trying to control different things out there
    Can only lead to deep despair
        Ultimately all I have power over is myself
        And if I don't exercise that power,
            I'll be lost, I will be lost.

I am worthy, you are worthy, too, we are all worthy,
    Says who? It must come from within,
        It must come from within,
            I am worthy, it must come from within, and
            You are worthy.
                It must come from within. It
                Must come from
                  Within.

THINKING

Without hope, it's impossible to cope
With the things that you have done.
Without faith, you can never escape
From the things you must overcome.

Are you tired of being caught in the
Clutches of your mind feeling like you
Might be running out of time, then
Tell me, what are you going to do?

You might want to change, change your thinking.
You have to be persistent, you might want
To change, change your thinking, determine
To be determined. Thinking, like a bulldog who won't let go.

You can't get rid of a harmful thought, if you think
You can, you're going to stay caught. Then what
Should you do with that harmful thought?
Exchange it for a helpful thought.

You see, your thoughts create your feelings,
Your feelings create you thoughts, do you want
To be healed? Or do you want to stay caught?
Change your thinking!

I CHOOSE LOVE

They say life is what you make it and I'm going
to make mine true.
It will be true love, love, love...
Each and every day no matter what you do or say, I'm going to
Choose love, love, true love

I know some days will be easier and some a little more difficult
It's still about love, love, true love and I choose love.
It's so nice to know that through all of life's ups and downs, I can
smile or wear a frown.

So I won't, let life bring or keep me down, I won't surrender, I
won't surrender.
And when I'm not in a loving space, I'll love by not doing any
harm to anyone in any way.
I will choose love, love, and true love.

FORGIVENESS

I believe in love, I believe in peace, and I choose,
I choose to forgive

forgive (forgive, forgive, forgive)
forgive (forgive, forgive)

All of this forgiving, tell me what's it all about?
I have done some things that I wish could be changed.
No matter how much I wish this, wishing it, it's all in vain.
The damage has been done and I can't change that.
No matter how much I want to, this is just a fact.

forgive (forgive, forgive, forgive)
forgive (forgive, forgive)

Although others may never forgive me for the things I've done.
Still I must learn to forgive those I feel hurt by
and those who cannot forgive me.
Most of all, I must learn to forgive myself

So much pain and suffering my actions have caused others.
You can't go back – you can't change that – it's just a fact.
So you're saying I can't do anybody any good if I keep looking
where I fell.
Got to get up – dust myself off and stop choosing to live in hell.
I believe in love, I believe in peace, and that's why I choose, I
choose to forgive.

PRELUDE TO *GIVE ME HOPE*

No matter how imperfect we may seem to be, I still believe that
every single person on this planet was born with something
special to contribute.

Somewhere within each of us, this special something is
priceless and as precious as a babies smile.

When the mentally ill are resurrected with hope and find their
voice, they then can rediscover and share with us the precious
gifts they brought to this world.
Please! Give us hope.

GIVE ME HOPE

Just trying to find some stillness, what's standing in the way?
Mental illness
You see peace keeps eluding me, if peace is real
someone help me find it
If I do or say something that is disturbing to you
Please don't talk down to me, remember the oath
that you took,
You swore, you swore to treat me with dignity

Give me hope no matter how small it may be
A little bit of hope might put me on the road to recovery
Give me hope—help me, help me, help me to heal my mind

It seems like every chance you get you want to put me down
It makes me sad and I feel so bad, when you wake up,
you will realize
When you treat me that way, you're putting both of us down
When you treat me that way, you're putting both of us down

I know you don't understand why I do what I do
Tell you the truth–sometimes I don't either,
I may not have it all figured out,
Please be patient, cause like you,
I'm doing the best that I can
Please give me some hope so I can feel better
And let this hell I'm living in come to an end

Give me hope—this illness has taken up so much of my time
Give me hope—hope gives me energy it strengthens my mind
Give me hope—no matter how small it might be
A little bit of hope might put me on the road to recovery

I'M READY TO FLY AGAIN

I'm ready to fly again
I'm ready to forgive my sins
I'm ready to fly again
It's a new beginning and not the end

I've been down too long
It's time to write a new chapter to this song
One of hope, love, and understanding
One of joy, peace, and forgiveness
One to let everybody know that it's okay to start again

Each day that I wake up
I'll say the words thank you
I'll pray for love in my thoughts, words, and actions
And if I fall short, I'll forgive myself and start again

I'm ready to fly again
I'm ready to forgive my sins
I'm ready to fly again
It's a new beginning and not the end

Epilogue

To My Children

      Looking back at my life and the consuming desire to help children and others who were suffering, combined with the incredible pain and paralyzing fear of my own childhood that I was carrying at the time, I was driven with unrelenting passion to help. This driving passion unknown to me at the time created a huge imbalance within me. I started having what is sometimes called *tunnel vision*. I was focused on one thing only, making lots of money to help children and others. I was totally obsessed with this mission.

      During this period I was unmarried and fathered several children. I was 18 when my first child was born. Ironically, while on this mission to help children, I was not there for you, my own children. At the same time it was very important to me to be seen in your eyes and in the eyes of my other family and friends as someone who was successful, as someone who had made it and had value.

      Unfortunately, although money can be used to do good things, this was not the most important thing you needed. You needed a dad who was in your life; I thought I would make it up to you when I so-called made it. I worked at music as though success was always just around the corner. *I'm almost there; I'm almost there.* Days, months, and years went by, but I was always *almost there.*

Looking back, a call on your birthdays, just a card or being there for the holidays, or making sure I was with you on your first day of school, things like that would have been far, far more precious and important to you and to me than becoming a "success." Even to this day I regret my choices about not participating in your lives. I know the past is the past and I can't change it, but if I could, with great joy, I most certainly would.

Instead of living a tunnel vision-type life, where everything was Now! Now! Now! I would have strived for a more balanced life. When I try to picture what that life would have looked like, first and foremost, I would have a steady job to pay the bills. That by itself would have kept me from feeling so desperate. I would get my rest, eat healthy, and have an exercise program. I would have pursued music part-time. Maybe I would have taken music courses and, who knows, maybe become a music teacher. Maybe I could have taught you to sing or play an instrument. As I do presently, every day and throughout the days I would give thanks to God and listen from within for my Higher Power's loving guidance.

My children, you are smart, attractive, and in your own individual ways successful. Just by the fact that you made something of yourselves in spite of not having a dad around shows your strength and character.

If I had the chance to do it all over again, I would be there for every birthday and when your first tooth fell out, tell you about the tooth fairy and the importance of putting that tooth under the pillow at night. Christmas would be a blast as I watch your anticipation and the excitement on your little faces and sparkling eyes just before the unwrapping of presents. Hugs would be a-plenty. I would help you with homework, attend school activities, protect you from harm, and play with you every chance I got. We would have gone on picnics, to the fair, hiking, and swimming.

Each morning I would greet you with something like, "How are you this morning with your wonderful self?" At night, while tucking you into bed, I can see myself reading or singing a song to precious you. I would be there to listen to your joys and sorrows, and constantly remind you of how so very special you are to me and the world.

You would know without any doubts that your father truly loves you so very deeply. And let's not forget, without any doubts, your boyfriends would have been under heavy scrutiny. It would have been fascinating to experience walking you down the aisle of marriage.

The most important thing I would have done would be to let you know about a God who loves you unconditionally and that this God not only lives within you, but can be found in everything and everywhere. God has a great purpose for your life. *You are not here by accident.* No matter how difficult it gets, know that God will see you through any and all adversities and situations. In some of my darkness moments, when I felt hopeless and helpless, God was there seeing me through it all even though I didn't know it or even believe it at the time. Pain and suffering is unavoidable. Through the pain and suffering I ultimately found a deeper peace and understanding that I would not otherwise have found. When the storms of life come into your lives, just hold on. Help is always there. Every single thing has a lesson to teach you. Always believe that. And, in the very end, it will always and only be, *God and you.*

I'm deeply sorry for not being there for you. I ask for your forgiveness.

With great love and respect,

Your dad

The End, for Now

Helpful Works and Media

Like most things that one reads, watches, or listens to, certain things make a positive impression on you, some don't, and some just go by you. Like I used to hear one person say from time to time, "Take what you can use here and leave the rest."

No matter how defeated we may feel (I have felt hopelessly defeated), there is a part in us that will never or can never give in to fears and intimidations. In various ways these references truly helped me to understand that fact. We have the choice of living a fear-based or love-based life. In the end only love—wanting the best for others and for one's self—brings us peace, joy, and contentment. These references are about authentic power (from within), courage, compassion, fearlessness, love, peace, understanding, forgiveness, and wisdom. I want these things more than anything else in this world.

Anatomy of an Epidemic: Magic Bullets, Psychiatric Drugs, and the Astonishing Rise of Mental Illness in America by Robert Whitaker. This book educated me on the history of medication and the pros and cons. This is a must read for all. Amazon.com gave it five stars. ❖

Deep & Simple by Bo Lozoff. For anyone whose goal is to become the best person they can be and to make their community and the world a better place, *Deep & Simple* without a doubt has the potential to help you reach those goals. This is not a twenty-first century get-fixed-quick book. I was struck by the author's simple but profound explanation about how to reach these goals. He explains the grave importance of communion with our inner light without ignoring our essential responsibilities to our community. ❖

Forgiveness Is a Choice: A Step-by-Step Process for Resolving Anger and Restoring Hope by Dr. Robert Enright. This is the book I used when studying forgiveness for the first time in a forgiveness group. It helped me to understand the power of forgiveness, if one chooses to forgive. This book will also teach the important steps involved in forgiving. ❖

The Four Agreements: A Practical Guide to Personal Freedom (A Toltec Wisdom Book) by Miguel Ruiz. This comes in book and audio CD. This is a nuts and bolts type book that really breaks things down. It's simplistic, and direct. It really helped me to understand the power of words and also the human condition in terms of how we got to be the way that we are, how to overcome it, and who *we all are*. I can't say enough about this book. ❖

Gratitude: A Way of Life by Louise L. Hay and friends was a lucky accident for me. Louise and her friends each share experiences about the importance of being grateful. Her friends are authors in their own right and have written books about the physical, mental, emotional, and spiritual issues of healing.

I had forgotten a book title and called the library for some help. The librarian read off a long list of titles but none of them rang a bell. Suddenly the title *Gratitude* jumped out at me. It wasn't the one I was looking for but I asked for it and I am so glad I did. The first few pages had me smiling. In fact, it's hard to even think about the book without smiling and sometimes even laughing. As I read on, the beauty of it drew tears of gratitude. This book couldn't have come into my life at a more perfect time.

In the *Gratitude* Louise Hay said, "When we live with grateful hearts, fear cannot enter, guilt is dissolved, and there is only peace, love, forgiveness, and understanding." I am ever so grateful that I have the opportunity to still do some good things in spite of myself. Those words, especially the word "understanding," help me to better understand why a part of me, because of my actions, will live out the remainder of my life, feeling a deep, intense sadness over the tremendous pain and suffering my actions have caused. Another part of me feels extremely grateful knowing in the clearest ways how I want to spend my remaining days on this earth. And that is being of help to others through writings, music, and maybe speaking on some level. On this more purposeful road I am now traveling, I have found and continue to find things that bring me great joy when it comes to being of service to others. ❖

Healing Trauma: Guided Imagery for Posttraumatic Stress by Belleruth Naparstek. This is a guided meditation CD that also uses powerful affirmations for healing trauma. As part of the heading says, "... not by reliving the trauma, but by metaphorically shifting it, incrementally over time with repeated listening." ❖

Inner and Outer Peace Through Meditation by Rajinder Singh. I come back to this guide time and time again and share it with anyone who will listen. Beginners and current practitioners can benefit from the sage advice and simple exercises. Of all the materials I suggest in this section, this book is my holy grail—the peace I have been seeking on my journey to heal and understand. I highly recommend it. ❖

Meditation to Help with Anger and Forgiveness by Belleruth Naparstek. This CD uses powerful affirmations to deal with the anger and bitterness that keeps one from a feeling of wellness and peace. All one has to do is listen to it repeatedly. It will do its work. ❖

The Power Is Within You by Louise L. Hay. This is a great title and a great book. I chose to listen to the CD version of this book. I found it inspirational, empowering, and true. ❖

The Power of FORGIVING by Everett L. Worthington, Jr., is a powerful easy to read little book and a great follow-up to the book *Forgiveness Is a Choice.* When one is ready, meaning in their own time, I believe the choice to forgive or not to forgive will be very obvious. ❖

The Power of Now: A Guide to Spiritual Enlightenment by Eckhart Tolle. The title says it. It's about the power and importance of learning to live in the present. I read this book about four years ago, and I'm in the process of rereading it. This book is just plain excellent. It's another one of those nuts and bolts type books. The past is gone and the future isn't here. I only have this moment and it just became the past. ❖

The Prophet by Kahlil Gibran. This book is a beautiful and poetic way of looking at life. I read this book as a teenager and recently reread it. If I could have practiced and understood back then what I understand presently, what a difference it could have made. They say knowledge is of no use if you don't use it. ❖

The Road Less Traveled by M Scott Peck (psychiatrist). In recently rereading this one, it helps me to understand even more the part my suffering played in my recovery process. Dr. Peck explains the importance of suffering and how it relates to mental illness, recovery, and spiritual growth. ❖

Search of the Self is a course that I have been exploring for over seventeen years. It totally goes against some of my early teachings about me being a sinner rather than me committing sins. I believe my tragedy and ending up in an institution played its part in me being open to the possibilities of these new and liberating teachings. This is where I was introduced to the teaching that captivated me that said blaming others had to stop and that I had to start taking responsibility for how I thought, felt, and acted. Now I know what real power is. ❖

The Seat of the Soul by Gary Zukav. In rereading this book after many years, it was like reading it for the first time. So many things illuminated my mind and heart. I don't mean to sound like a broken record but this is another one of those excellent reads. ❖

Take These Broken Wings by Daniel Mackler. This feature length DVD documentary is about two extraordinary individuals who recovered from severe schizophrenia without medication. A friend of mine said after watching it that "the evidence is irrefutable." ❖

A Way Out of Madness by Daniel Mackler and Matthew Morrissey. It's about the key to recovery from mental illness, the important role of family, and powerful personal stories.

Contributors include:
- Patch Adams, M.D., who was the inspiration for the Robin Williams film.
- Joanne Greenberg, author, *I Never Promised You a Rose Garden.*
- David Oaks, director, Mind Freedom International Will Hall, co-founder, Freedom Center. ❖

We're All Doing Time by Bo Lozoff. This book came across my path only recently, and I consider it an outstanding addition to my resources for improving how I do my life. On the one hand, the book gives very specific how-to advice on topics such as keeping food simple and doing breathing exercises. For the last two months I used some of the breathing techniques demonstrated in the book. Mentally and emotionally I feel much more peaceful. I can't tell you how great and reassuring that feels.

On the other hand, the book explores themes of love, compassion, and forgiveness—the same qualities Bo taught and exemplified during his decades of work with thousands of men and women inmates. The second half of the book shares letters written to Bo and his responses to those letters. Reading these letters, although sometimes tragic and extremely sad, confirmed my deep belief not only in a loving spirit within us all but also how much we are all alike. As one of the credits said, "This wonderful book helps connect us all."

Wait until you read what these prisoners have to say. If these letters don't give you hope, then I just don't know about you. The letters let you know that people can change no matter their circumstances. The book also tells how to play a crucial part in making this a better world for others and for yourself. The book will expand your understanding of the connectedness of people and show how you can be the gentle caring messenger who gives another person the potential to change. I say potential because in the end it is always up to each of us to decide for ourselves to change or not to change. Bo said, trying to make big changes is almost impossible, but the small changes possible in the small moments are what eventually lead to the big changes. He said let's say that I have been a thief all of my life and now I want to change. I'm thinking about taking something. In that moment of thinking about that, I can choose not to do it. If I'm sincere, honest, and bulldog determined about changing, it won't be about will I make it, it will be about making it *that* moment. You've heard the saying that life by the yard is hard and life by the inch is a cinch.

My 2015 New Year's resolution was to not let negative thinking about others come out my mouth. This is a resolution that does not depend on others. Nearing the end of April 2015 I give myself an A minus. I definitely feel more peaceful, stronger emotionally, and more confident, which motivates me to stick with it because there's no doubt in my mind that I'm on the right path. In the book it lists different prayers and I found the perfect one to assist me in my goal of not speaking badly of others.

When you are ready and in your own time, you will be thankful for a book like this. The honesty is so incredibly beautiful. Thank you Bo. And thank you, Sita, for carrying on his and your precious work. In 2012, loving, compassionate, kind, and courageous Bo was in a motorcycle accident and is no longer physically with us. His Human Kindness Foundation continues. Books and CDs are free for inmates at Human Kindness Foundation, P.O. Box 61619, Durnham, North Carolina 27715. I truly enjoyed writing about this book. ❖

Wherever You Go There You Are by Kabat-Zinn. I read this book very early on in my recovery journey. The seed this book planted in me was that no matter where I physically went, I couldn't get away from myself. And, my problems are not outside of me but inside. That meant I was going to have to face and solve them from within. No avoiding, trying to hide, or running away was going to work because wherever I go there I am. ❖

Wishes Fulfilled and *Religious Point of View* and other PBS-TV broadcasts by Wayne Dyer were initially difficult for me to get a grip on. My ego kept some of his words of wisdom from entering me. I'm thankful that some of his teachings got through anyway. As my ego has been shrinking through the years, I found myself appreciating his wonderful, powerful teachings so much more. All of his teachings tell it like it is. Whatever I heard, read or saw of his teachings, it helped me with transforming my life. ❖

One Last Note about Works and Media

One problem I discovered about writing a book is that it is never really finished. Life and learning keep happening. I keep wanting to add one more thing, and I keep thinking that maybe this word or that word is better. I worry that sometimes I expressed myself in a way that was too harsh, or I softened something and so wasn't accurate to the facts or true to myself.

This is how it is in the Helpful Works and Media chapter, too. I keep finding one more essential book that simply has to be added. So the book was done — even the proofs were done. And, yes, I did find another book that I just had to tell you about. It's Marianne Williamson's *A Return to Love: Reflections on the Principles of A Course in Miracles* (1992). Funny thing is that I was led to Ms. Williamson's book by a quote that I always thought was by President Nelson Mandela. "Our deepest fear is not that we are powerful beyond measure. It is our light, not our darkness, that most frightens us." She said that in her book. Find it; get it; read it. Okay. I'm done now. Maybe.

Acknowledgements

THANK YOU!

I am thankful for everyone I have ever met or known because in some way through them, because of them, I was given the opportunity to grow in some way. Through those experiences, pleasant or not so pleasant, I've learned about my strengths and weaknesses as I continue to learn and grow.

I am thankful for the institution that kept me safe and allowed me to write this book.

I am thankful for the National Empowerment Center for empowering me with knowledge and understanding

I am thankful for and have learned about the importance of my family and great friends who love and care about me in spite of myself. Without their loving support, recovery would have been almost if not impossible.

I am thankful for one of my peers who took the time to use his creativity to come up with the picture of a bird to symbolize my finding my wings.

I am grateful to the busy people who gave the gift of their time to read early versions of my manuscript and offer valuable suggestions. They helped make my book more complete. And I am thankful for my sister and my friend who gave their time and attention to read the almost finished version. The book is more complete and more polished because of them.

I wish I had a way to look ahead so I could thank the friends and family who help spread the word that this book is out there. I'm thanking you all right now anyway.

I am thankful for my editor. When my editor came to meet me through a friend of a friend for the first time, I automatically sensed that this is the right person to help me with my book. My editor has been professional, kind, gentle, patient, encouraging, insightful, and so very understanding. And without question, the right one.

Most of all I am thankful for love. To give up on love is to live a hopeless life forever groping around in the dark. To give up on love is to give up on others and myself. I am so thankful for love.

Notes